Baby Steps

Baby Steps

How Lesbian Alternative Insemination
Is Changing the World

Amy Agigian

WESLEYAN UNIVERSITY PRESS
Middletown, Connecticut

Published by Wesleyan University Press,
Middletown, CT 06459

© 2004 by Amy Agigian

All rights reserved.

Printed in the United States of America

Library of Congress Cataloging-in-
Publication Data
Agigian, Amy.
Baby steps : how lesbian alternative insemi-
nation is changing the world / Amy Agigian.
    p.   cm.
Includes bibliographical references and index.
ISBN 0-8195-6629-2 (cloth : alk. paper)
    1. Lesbian mothers—United States.
    2. Lesbian mothers—Legal status, laws,
etc.—United States. 3. Self-insemination—
United States. 4. Self-insemination—Social
aspects. I. Title.
HQ75.53.A45 2004
306.874'3'08664—dc22   2004002036

I dedicate this book to my mother
Judith Linda Agigian
and to my son
Max Jude Agigian

Contents

Preface

I started paying serious attention to lesbian alternative insemination (AI) in the 1980s. At that time, we were already in the midst of the lesbian baby boom, and AI was the method of choice for many lesbian families. Since then, a great deal has changed.

The medical establishment has changed.[1] Fifteen years ago, doctors had a monopoly on medical AI, including access to sperm banks, and almost without exception denied access to lesbians. Lesbians were excluded from medical AI by doctors' heterosexism.[2] For example, when I moved to Boston in the late 1980s, lesbians could receive insemination services at only two places. Only one small sperm bank in the country catered to lesbians and unmarried heterosexual women.[3]

While once physicians reigned supreme and were gatekeepers over medical care, today they have lost much of their power. The rise of Health Management Organizations (HMOs) and managed care in general has weakened physician hegemony over medicine. Physicians' decisions are constrained, or at least strongly influenced, by the policies of third-party payers, without whose approval the physician will not get paid. More and more doctors are employed by others—whether hospitals, HMOs, or the government—whose policies often limit their role as gatekeepers. (These policies still often coincide with the physician's own reluctance to provide infertility services for lesbians.) The sea change away from physician hegemony, sometimes called "the proletarianization of physicians,"[4] allows unprecedented access to infertility services, including AI, for lesbians who can pay. This change has not lessened the medicalization and social control of the body, but rather shifted its locus.

Today, not one medical practice in Boston will deny a client insemination services because she is a lesbian. That does not mean that clients are treated equally well in every setting. Far from it. But even practices that have a reputation for being lesbian-*unfriendly* will say they welcome all clients regardless of sexual orientation. This change is occurring unevenly and varies by location. Many U.S. physicians still refuse to inseminate lesbians.

Another change is that lesbian AI has become professionalized and medicalized. Early in the lesbian baby boom, it was understood that AI was a simple, low-tech process that could be performed at home with materials you already have around the house (e.g., a turkey baster and mason jar). A friend, acquaintance, or friend of a friend contributed semen. The only mediation between sperm donor and inseminator was a possible friend or other courier to maintain anonymity when desired. In tune with the women's health movement, lesbians seeking insemination were skeptical and critical of the male-dominated medical establishment. A guiding ethos was self-empowerment and self-help, specifically outside of the domain of paternalistic doctors.

Today, lesbians almost always practice AI in a way that is both high-tech and professionally mediated. The AIDS epidemic provoked the norm of medical screenings for potential sperm donors, as well as the norm of freezing and quarantining semen until its donor gets a second negative HIV test result.[5] While inseminating lesbians used to use the lower-tech process of charting their fertility with a thermometer and by changes in cervical mucous, today they are more likely to use a commercial ovulation-predictor kit, or even transvaginal ultrasounds. Early in the baby boom, lesbians were more likely to enlist people in their social circle as sperm donors, while today they are more likely to go through a sperm bank. Lesbians once inseminated at home, while today they are more likely to inseminate in the doctor's office or clinic. Most lesbians previously inseminated by placing the semen in their own vaginas or having their lover do it, while today many lesbians opt for intra-uterine insemination (IUI), which must be performed by a medically trained professional. In sum, today's lesbians use the full gamut of infertility industry resources, from boutique sperm to in vitro fertilization. This medicalization can be taken as a sign of lesbian liberation, co-optation, or both.

The U.S. legal situation has also changed, albeit more slowly. Fifteen years ago, the law in most jurisdictions had never heard of lesbian AI, and lesbians had scanty legal mechanisms for protecting the integrity of their families. Today, family law remains largely heterosexist and patriarchal,[6] notwithstanding a growing tendency to allow people to privately negotiate the terms of their familial relationships.[7] However, those lesbians who can afford it, in a small number of U.S. jurisdictions, can implement significant legal protections for their families, including second-parent adoption. In numerous other developed countries, the law has changed just as quickly.

Lesbian discourses and practices of AI have also changed, as once-marginalized activities have become more normalized, bureaucratized, and, some would say, co-opted. Lesbian AI emerged in the context of the lesbian-feminist movement of the late 1960s and 1970s. It was practiced originally by lesbian feminists, including lesbian separatists. For these women, having children without men was often a political as well as a personal act, and anonymous donors were often preferred. Today, the right to marriage is high on the lesbian political agenda, and a sense of entitlement to the rights afforded to heterosexual couples is a dominant ethos among inseminating lesbians. The psychosocial importance of sperm donors to their children is an important consideration for the large number of inseminating lesbians who choose, or wish to choose, known sperm donors.[8] Many choose gay men as sperm donors and negotiate a limited familial relationship with them.

These transformations in lesbian insemination practices have many causes. In addition to those mentioned above, one of the most important is that the infertility industry has consolidated, and lesbians have been recognized as a lucrative market. Lesbians are no longer excluded from infertility medicine. In many cases they are courted. Because health insurance generally will not cover lesbian AI, lesbians must pay out of pocket, and therefore at higher rates than insurance companies would reimburse. Techniques such as intracytoplasmic sperm injection (ICSI) have been developed that enable once-infertile men to become biological fathers, thus reducing the market for AI.[9] In the struggle between capitalist imperatives and heterosexist prohibitions, the balance seems to be tipping toward the almighty dollar, with lesbian dollars increasingly welcomed.

The rapidly changing state of lesbian AI can itself be seen as a symptom of our ultramodern era and lesbians' incorporation into its circuits of operation.[10] A key characteristic of ultramodernity is speed-up, which most of us experience as the rapid pace of life: hectic schedules, mind-body stress, lack of sleep, and/or near-constant demands. This speed-up is related to the ascendance of communication technologies that bombard us with telelectronic stimulus, where information multiplies faster than anyone can possibly use or even decipher it, and where we are increasingly "wired" and therefore accessible to all kinds of others, known and unknown, personal and corporate, wanted and unwanted. Ultramodernity also entails the transformation of everything possible into a code that can be "known," manipulated, and made profitable at dizzying rates.[11] The effort to "know" and dominate beings and things alike is advanced through the profitable area of genetic research. In this explosion of data, even those activities that were formerly sites of resistance to domination can become digitalized and repackaged for consumption. Capitalism has become liquid on many levels. Inseminating lesbians, particularly those who use sperm banks, are among the beneficiaries of this ultramodern turn in genetics, family, medicine, and law. I argue that ultramodernity is a key concept for understanding the complex contours of lesbian AI.

This rapid state of change also makes it difficult to write a book that is up to date, and impossible to write one that will remain up to date.[12] Still, I hope to do justice to some of the incredibly complex issues that inhere to lesbian AI, and to provide a sense of the challenge and accommodation, love and anger, radicalism and conservatism, creativity and chutzpah that characterize lesbian AI.

My analysis has changed along with these historical changes. Questions that seemed crucial to me ten years ago have become stale. Others have arisen in their place. I have made peace with a number of practices—medical and social—that seemed unbearable in the past, and have come to question practices that once seemed liberating. And I am finding race and class to be as salient to lesbian AI as sexuality and gender.

This book builds on solid empirical research showing that lesbian mothers are at least as good for their children as heterosexual mothers. This conclusion has been reached repeatedly in social-scientific studies over the past twenty-five years.[13] Legal scholar David L. Chambers presents a good encapsulation of the research:

> Researchers who compared children raised in lesbian and heterosexual households found few or no differences in the development of gender identity, gender-role behavior, or sexual orientation. Studies have also found no deficits among children of lesbian mothers in other aspects of personal development, including separation-individuation, locus of control, self-concept, intelligence, or moral judgment. In addition, numerous studies have shown that children raised by lesbians have normal, healthy relationships with other children as well as with adults.[14]

I feel no need to present the voluminous research regarding lesbians' fitness as mothers. Instead, I submit that all ideas to the contrary (and they are legion) are based not in fact but in prejudice. For the purposes of this book, the fitness of lesbian mothers is a given.[15]

I try to avoid making generalizations about lesbians who use/d AI, and instead honor and acknowledge their diversity. Lesbian mothers who have used AI, like all mothers, are distinct individuals, with particular histories, personalities, demographics, and names. Each one faces different challenges and opportunities on the life-path that includes lesbian identity, insemination, and motherhood. Even social forces such as sexism and heterosexism, with which all contend, are not monolithic entities that affect each woman in the same way.

While I make an effort to note when my argument applies to other groups as well, this book centers on lesbian insemination in the United States. Lesbian AI in the San Francisco Bay Area occupies a particularly prominent place, both because of my own connections there and since so many of the authors and organizations engaged with these issues are there. Lesbian AI is a transnational phenomenon, however, and I discuss research from some two dozen countries. This book is an institutional critique, not an ethnographic study of intentional lesbian families. I specifically do not seek to "explore" or specularize intentional lesbian mothers.[16] Rather than making inseminating lesbians and/or their families into objects of study, I interrogate the institutional forces with which these families must contend. While no case is typical, and no one's life is collapsible into general narratives, powerful institutional discourses affect everyone. The medical establishment, while hardly static or monolithic, is a major institution of social control with which nearly everyone (including intentional lesbian mothers) must contend. The law, even if we never run afoul of it, shapes all of our lives in concrete and pervasive ways. And normative notions of the family haunt attempts to live outside their bounds. I critically map the conflicts surrounding AI by juxtaposing lesbian, medical, and legal discourses, articulating the high stakes that drive the often-contesting parties. By problematizing the institutional discourses, rather than their targets, I make a political claim about where the (social) problem lies. The concept of discourse, for me, is a way of talking about the power of different ways to describe reality, and of being in reality through language. Discourse is not a system in which ideas descend from top down, but rather one in which powerful stories proliferate, and potentially subversive ones coexist and conflict with dominant ones. I hope to be able to show this complexity in lesbian AI. Lesbians participate in conventional discourses at the same time as they generate discourses that resist their own domination and domestication.

While discourses may be analyzed textually, they also have powerful material effects on people's lives. For instance, while the law is discursive, it also has the coercive power of the state behind it.[17] Legal scholar Ruthann Robson writes,

> Lesbians experience . . . concrete manifestations of [the law's] violence daily: we are more likely to be imprisoned than heterosexual women, we lose property in courts that do not recognize our relationships, and we have our children removed. . . . Such expressions of concrete violence are supported by the law's symbolic violence in discourse.[18]

Biomedicine is also discursive, and it wields enormous (legally sanctioned) material power over our lives. Medical personnel and objects limit, incite, and penetrate our most intimate bodily and psychic selves. In their most extreme exercise of power, people with medical authority may subject us to psychiatric incarceration and psychopharmacological "treatments" as well as the (medicalized) death penalty. Insurance policy discourses may grant or deny us reproductive services as well as life-saving medical treatments. They may also prevent, or consign us to, (medical-expense related) bankruptcy, and ultimately, poverty.

Families are discursive, yet they too operate with vast material power by and over their members. Infants and children experience literally life-or-death dependence on their caretakers. Equally profound, the inner life of family members may be nurtured or crushed by the great power of other family members whose latitude is supported by both custom and law.

Where I Am Coming From

My own relationship to lesbian AI is many-sided. My mother came out as a lesbian when I was ten years old. My sister and I were raised in a lesbian household, in a rather politicized lesbian-feminist community, for five years, until just before my mother's untimely death at thirty-eight (which is my age as I write this). During those five years, I became sensitized to lesbian and feminist issues, and familiar with a slice of (mostly white, suburban) lesbian life. I started identifying as bisexual when I was about fifteen, when I had moved in with my father and his collective household in Berkeley. I left that house after less than a year, and sustained myself with a variety of jobs and a small monthly Social Security check, combined with the relative largesse of my boyfriend, who was a housepainter. I was acutely aware of the differences between most of my high school classmates and myself in family and economic status. Spending my late teenaged years with no parents, moving several times a year, and working low-paid jobs (mostly in restaurants) all helped make me the sociologist I have become.

At eighteen, I moved to Santa Cruz to attend the University of California, and I immersed myself in its vibrant lesbian community. In both Santa Cruz and the greater Bay Area, I knew numerous lesbians who had conceived their children with AI. The oldest of these children whom I knew personally were born in the early 1980s, and people around me were inseminating frequently. I was aware of a variety of creative parenting arrangements. Besides the typical two-mommies-and-their-babies norm, I knew a handful of cases where more than half a dozen lesbians (who had various relationships with each other) agreed to be co-mothers of a single baby conceived and birthed by one of them.

Although sometimes the babies with more than three or four doting mothers seemed a little spoiled, and despite my own less-than-idyllic experiences with my lesbian stepmother, I supported lesbian family arrangements absolutely (and still do). Male-dominated families had had their chance, and bungled it badly, as many people I knew agreed readily. Women having the opportunity to parent without men seemed to me an important procreative freedom, especially for lesbians. I took a part-time job as an anonymous sperm courier for an AI program geared toward lesbians. My responsibilities varied over the next several years as I worked to facilitate the pregnancy, and ensure the privacy, of the program's participants.

I met sperm donors in parking lots, parks, and their homes, and relieved them of small containers that I placed immediately into the crook of my armpit. I handed cash to anonymous men, some of whose faces were still flushed, in exchange for a small warm vial. I pulled frozen semen vials from a tank, and thawed them in my hands until I could draw their contents into a syringe to present to a client.

I responded to late night phone calls from women whose ovulatory status required insemination the next morning. Sometimes I delivered semen "on ice" to clients who wanted to inseminate at home. Occasionally I drove for hours with semen wrapped in a temperature-controlled gel pack to meet a woman waiting for me at her home. I drove many times with a fresh vial nestled between my legs, to keep it at the optimal temperature.

On many mornings I unlocked an office in the early hours for a woman, or a couple, whom I let into an examining room to prepare for insemination. I pulled the sterile paper down over the table with the stirrups and laid out a gown. In the next room, I put on latex gloves, opened individually-packaged surgical syringes (which I carried in my car's glove box), removed the needles and disposed of them in biohazard containers. I drew the semen into two (or, much more rarely, three) syringes, and presented them in a clean paper towel to the waiting woman. I made chitchat with the women or even little jokes about the moon or the auspicious amount of semen in "this batch." Back in the next room I turned on the radio and timed my wait, then knocked on the woman's door and said "it's been twenty minutes." I took her payment.

I privately celebrated the joyous news of conceptions and of ensuing births. I felt awful, and sometimes irrationally guilty, for the women who, after a heroic amount of effort, finally quit trying. I tried to respect everyone's privacy and always to forget the names, faces, addresses, and voices of both clients and donors.

And all of these hours were dwarfed by the time I spent thinking: thinking and talking, thinking and reading, thinking and writing, about what in the world it all meant. These experiences deeply informed my thinking and the lines of questioning that evolved first into my doctoral dissertation in sociology and then into this book.

Later, as a graduate student, I co-organized and co-taught the first Lesbian and Gay Studies classes at Brandeis University. I assumed that if I ever decided to have children, they would be conceived with AI. I had a robust lesbian identity, and was immersed in lesbian and queer theory, film, literature, and politics. Today, I am a junior member of the Sociology faculty at Suffolk University in Boston, where my teaching focuses on women's issues. I am once again bisexual, and maintain a strong connection to the lesbian, gay, bisexual, and transgender world. I am the blessed and stressed mother of a young son, and my (male) partner is a stay-at-home dad.

All of these parts of my biography (and surely many more) have influenced the creation of this book.

This book contains two appendixes. One describes my methodology, which is strongly influenced by Gerald Vizenor's concept of "socio-acupuncture."[19] The other contains definitions and discussions of several key terms used throughout the book. Interested readers are encouraged to read this material before proceeding any further. Others may want to save it for later or even skip it entirely. Now, welcome to the rest of the book!

Acknowledgments

It is a pleasure to be able to thank some of the generous souls whose help has made the completion of this book possible.

While working on this project, I received invaluable support from many kind souls: I thank Haig Agigian, Laura Michele Agigian, Jane Benson, Janet Brooks, Candace Carey, Sara Carleton, Olivia Cheever, Patsy Cobb, Trevor "Coconut" Cralle, Ronny "Spacecraft Lurch Moonward" Crawford, Ann Davidson, Elise Ficarra, Ghassan Haddad, the late and much missed Marcia Hood-Brown, Sharon Jacques, Clara Lanyi, Frank Leone, JoAnn Loulan, Samuel Lurie, Maureen MacCarthy and Tori Smith, Grace Moore, Judy Music, Nora Nicosia, the late and much missed Joey Nicosia, Judy Panitch, Sharon Panitch and Rick Hecht, Rachel Roth, Nick Rubashkin and Drew Banks, Christine Sanni and Karen Seif, Marsha Saxton, Jenny Miller Sechler, Cory and Amanda Skuldt, Roger Solomon, Bob Stickgold, Elena Stone, Russell "Rusty" Weston, Ammie White, Anita Tishman Winkler, and Jennifer Yanco.

My thanks also go out to those who have critiqued chapters or the whole manuscript. Karen "SMD" Adler, Toni Amato, Melissa Bass, Will Brooke-DeBock, Teresa Brennan, Woody Brooks, Peter Conrad, Benjamin Davidson, Martha Denney, Ross Ellenhorn, Karen Hansen, Robbie Pfeufer Kahn, Cameron Macdonald, Lisa Nash, Stephen Pfohl, Catherine Rice, Nicholas Rubashkin, Tristan Taormino, Jennifer Trimble, Lauri Umanski, and several anonymous readers have all been generous with their time and critical skills.

I would like to acknowledge the mentoring and collegial support at Brandeis University of Shulamit Reinharz, Maury Stein, Stefan Timmermans, and the late and much missed Irving Kenneth Zola. At the Women's Studies Program Working Papers Series at Brandeis University, I thank Sarita Bhalotra, Andrea Most, Naomi Myrvaagnes, and Jo Anne Preston.

It has been wonderful to have a small group of colleagues also working on lesbian AI. For this pleasure I thank Susan Kahn, Laura Mamo, Lisa Jean Moore, and Maureen Sullivan.

Anne Pollock was the ideal research assistant: meticulous, level-headed, canny, and delightful. will get a special place in heaven for her eleventh-hour editorial aid. Annette Oliveira, my son's Nana/Abuelita, was extremely generous with her awesome editorial skills; when I could no longer look at the manuscript without screaming, Annette read every word with loving ruthlessness. Lyndsay Agans spent hours helping prepare the manuscript for publication. Suzanna Tamminen at Wesleyan

University Press has shepherded me through the process of book writing with grace and humor. All mistakes, of course, are mine alone.

Several institutions have been nurturing and challenging spaces, which have fostered my intellectual and personal development. Communities I have been privileged to be a part of include Maybeck High School, the U.C. Santa Cruz Women's Studies Department, Brandeis University Sociology Department, Brandeis University Women's Studies Program, Harvard University Committee on Degrees in Women's Studies, the Boston Women's Health Book Collective, and Suffolk University College of Arts and Science.

Suffolk University has been a nurturing and collegial space for intellectual work. Many thanks to the Suffolk Sociology Department as a whole, and especially to my close neighbors Carolyn Boyes-Watson, Sharon Kurtz, Jim Ptacek, and Felicia Wiltz. For collegial friendship I also want to thank my Suffolk comrades Kris Bursik, Kathleen Grathwol, Melissa Haussman, Marjorie Salvodon, and Lauri Umanski and the entire Women's and Gender Studies community.

I want to thank the extraordinary students I've had at Brandeis, Harvard, and Suffolk, especially those in "Reclaiming Bodies, Remapping Power: Lesbian and Gay Social Theories" at Brandeis, and those in "Women in Contemporary Society" at Suffolk. I am grateful that I was able to present pieces of my research on lesbian AI in a variety of academic forums and receive valuable feedback from a larger collegial community. I presented pieces of this work at meetings of the American Sociological Association, the Society for the Study of Social Problems, "Queer Sites: Bodies at Work, Bodies at Play: Studies in Lesbian and Gay Cultures," and MIT's Lecture Series: "The Politics and Technology of Motherhood."

I would also like to extend my sincere thanks to five exceptional women who have provided me with feminist collegiality, mentoring, and employment: Judy Norsigian, Shulamit Reinharz, Juliet Schor, Alexandra Todd, and Andrea Walsh.

On a more personal note, I give thanks to my parents and grandparents for working so hard to give me opportunities in life; I also acknowledge the hard work of so many parents who are unable, in spite of that work, to provide a better life for their children. I give thanks to the precious waters of our planet, especially that stretch of Pacific coastline between Pacifica and Santa Cruz. I am also grateful for the wonderful animals we share the Earth with—without these magical creatures my life would be bereft. In particular, my cats Chicklet and the late and much missed Sweet Pea helped me greatly during the process of writing this book, and taught me much about what it means to be human.

Thank you sweet Max, for giving me the gift of your Self.

For unstinting, creative, saintly support in editing and in life, I thank my mate, Bob Defandorf. More than anyone else, he has helped me make this the book I want it to be.

Finally, I want to thank those who have made the lesbian baby boom a reality, and those who have celebrated, supported, learned from, and fought for them. May we all live in peace and justice.

Abbreviations

AAP:	American Academy of Pediatrics
AATB:	American Association of Tissue Banks
ACOG:	American College of Obstetricians and Gynecologists
AFS:	American Fertility Society
AI:	alternative insemination; artificial insemination
AID:	alternative insemination by donor
AIDS:	Acquired Immune Deficiency Syndrome
AIH:	alternative insemination by husband
AIP:	artificial insemination with partner's sperm
AMA:	American Medical Association
APA:	American Psychiatric Association
ART:	assisted reproductive technology
ASRM:	American Society for Reproductive Medicine
BWHBC:	Boston Women's Health Book Collective
CDCP:	Centers for Disease Control and Prevention
CEDAW:	The (United Nations) Convention on the Elimination of All Forms of Discrimination against Women
CMV:	cytomegalovirus
COLAGE:	Children of Lesbians and Gays Everywhere
CRC:	The (United Nations) Convention on the Rights of the Child
DI:	Donor Insemination

DOMA:	The Defense of Marriage Act
GED:	General Educational Development
GIFT:	gamete intrafallopian transfer
HIV:	Human Immunodeficiency Virus
ICI:	intracervical insemination
ICSI:	intracytoplasmic sperm injection
IFFS:	International Federation of Fertility Societies
IGLHRC:	International Gay and Lesbian Human Rights Commission
IGLPA:	International Gay and Lesbian Parenting Association
IUI:	intrauterine insemination
IVF:	in vitro fertilization
IVI:	intravaginal insemination
LGBT:	lesbian, gay, bisexual, and transgender
NCLR:	National Center for Lesbian Rights
NGLTF:	National Gay and Lesbian Task Force
NIH:	National Institutes of Health
NLFS:	National Lesbian Family Study
NRT:	new reproductive technologies
NSFG:	National Survey of Family Growth
OB/GYN:	obstetrician/gynecologist; obstetrics/gynecology
OPK:	ovulation-prediction kit
OTA:	Office of Technology Assessment (of the U.S. Congress)
PIVMO:	penis in vagina with male orgasm
PQP:	prospective queer parents
PRS:	Pacific Reproductive Services
SCD:	semen collection device
SI:	self-insemination
TDI:	therapeutic donor insemination
TSBC:	The Sperm Bank of California
UDHR:	Universal Declaration of Human Rights
WHO:	World Health Organization
WRN:	Women's Rights Network
ZIFT:	zygote intrafallopian transfer

Baby Steps

I

Introduction

FROM SMALL THINGS, MAMA,

BIG THINGS ONE DAY COME.

— *Bruce Springsteen*

ABSTRACT

As the twentieth century began to unfold, the word "family" conjured images of Dad, the leader and provider, Mom, the nurturer and follower, and children who were to be seen and not heard. One hundred plus years have wrought myriad changes, which challenge this supposedly "normal" vision of family. Lesbian alternative insemination (AI) exists at the crossroads of three of the most controversial alternatives to the male-headed nuclear family: single motherhood, gay parenthood, and non-traditional procreation. Because it inhabits this flash point, lesbian AI is a rich practice through which to explore shifts in contemporary kinship arrangements. Alternative insemination, as thousands of lesbians now practice it, is unprecedented in both its means of conception and in the family forms it enables. Lesbian AI therefore brings into sharp relief some of our most taken-for-granted assumptions about families.

Alternative insemination, surrogate motherhood, and in vitro fertilization are now common forms of procreation. The families they help create symbolically rupture our traditional understandings of baby-making, motherhood, fatherhood, and sex. New forms of procreation may evoke ambivalence. They also compel us to examine our values, beliefs, anxieties, and dreams about the familial, intimate, and technological worlds we inhabit. Lesbian mothers and their families often redefine the traditional terms used to describe families. In this book, I discuss the effects of lesbian AI on three of the most powerful social institutions in U.S. society: medicine, law, and the family. My argument is twofold.

First, lesbian AI radically challenges the power structure, assumptions, and presumed "naturalness" of major social institutions.[1] Lesbian AI promotes gender and familial practices that are less sexist and less naturalized, and which move discourses around the family and gender in the direction of fluidity, hybridity, feminism, and choice.[2] By challenging core heteropatriarchal definitions of reality, lesbian AI can disrupt and refigure some of the foundations of society and psyche alike.[3] Lesbian AI thus contributes to a more democratic, tolerant, and just society.

At the same time, lesbian insemination is being recuperated back into traditional discourses of family, medicine, and the law. As it is co-opted, lesbian insemination strengthens the status quo of commercial culture, conservative family values, class-based legal and medical norms, and biomedicalized understandings of body and kinship. It also reinforces stratification both among lesbians and in the larger society.

Lesbian AI is unique among modes of procreation because it enables women to create families with no legal or psychological father, and because it involves the commercialization of men's procreative capacities rather than women's. Lesbian appropriation of medical technology (AI) that was intended to shore up nuclear families engenders quite different issues from use of the same technology by married or even unmarried heterosexual women.

Lesbian AI has transformed patriarchal cultural tropes across fields of social practice such as law, psychology, medicine, and kinship. In these fields, the invisibility that characterizes lesbian existence confronts the invisibility of patriarchal norms that suffuse society. In this confrontation, both are made visible. Lesbians, of course, are not "actually" invisible, but their existence and lives often disappear from sight since they are not represented (except sensationalistically) in most cultures, and since many heterosexuals assume that everyone else is heterosexual too. The "naturalness" of heteropatriarchal social arrangements (e.g., heteronormative motherhood, family, sexuality[4]) is strained by this exposure, revealing these arrangements as heavily regulated constructs. Paradoxically, the law of the fathers becomes visible at its moment of imposition. And contradictory pressures for and against visibility come to bear on lesbians who use AI.

Kinship forms enabled by lesbian AI disrupt three of the most powerful social institutions in our lives: medicine, the law, and the male-headed nuclear family. Each of these three, enmeshed with individual practices and played out in powerful institutions, profoundly affects inseminating lesbians and their families. Lesbian AI, intentionally or not, radically challenges the gendered social-control functions of these institutions, even while it replicates elements of heteropatriarchal kinship norms. Laws and regulations that address AI in most countries are based on the assumption of a nuclear family and thus fail to protect the integrity of intentional lesbian families.[5] Psychological and psychoanalytic theories likewise insist on the primacy of the father or phallus as an organizing principle in the psychosexual development of both girls and boys. Medical protocols define AI within a discourse of heteronormative "fertility medicine." Lesbian discourses, on the other hand, posit theories that are usually mother-centered and lesbian-friendly, and that aim to support the well being of family members without the intervention of male power.[6] These distinctive characteristics render lesbian AI unintelligible under existing theoretical frameworks used to discuss other forms of contractual and technological procreation.

I offer here a theory that makes this new form of family-making intelligible. I want to argue for legal, medical, and discursive (political) strategies that will empower the great majority of lesbians and their families, not only those with the most socioeconomic privilege. I seek openings for progressive social change, social justice, and the exercise of lesbians' human rights.

Lesbian AI

Alternative insemination is a process by which a woman attempts to achieve pregnancy through the non-coital introduction of sperm into her uterus. Intravaginal AI has been used in Europe and North America as a "treatment" for male infertility of married, moneyed, heterosexual couples for more than a century.

Insemination was (and in most cases still is) performed by physicians in their offices or infertility clinics, often with the sperm of anonymous men. Since the first commercial semen bank opened in the United States in 1972, semen banks have become a booming business.

How many sperm banks exist, what portion serve lesbians, and their average costs are difficult to discern. Fifty-nine sperm banks in all regions of the country are listed at SpermBankDirectory.com.[7] The insemination industry was estimated in 1987 to bring in about $160 million dollars a year in the United States alone.[8]

The use of AI has been documented in dozens of countries, rich and poor, and on every continent.[9] The most recent figures of the Office of Technology Assessment (OTA) of the U.S. Congress were gathered during a one-year period in 1986 and 1987. They estimated that 172,000 U.S. women underwent alternative insemination in 1986 to 1987, resulting in 35,000 births from alternative insemination by husband (AIH), and 30,000 births from alternative insemination by donor (AID).[10] In the United Kingdom, where better records are kept, 8,096 women underwent AI in 1994, resulting in the births of 1,085 babies. In France, it is estimated that 20,250 cycles of AI were carried out in 1991 (we do not know how many women these cycles were distributed among), resulting in 1,777 babies.[11] Conservatively, tens of thousands of children are conceived through AI each year. Since this has been so for at least fifteen years, approximately half a million to a million people now walk the Earth that were conceived with AI.[12]

Unless a doctor has his or her own source of semen, or the recipient brings her own sperm provider, frozen sperm is purchased from a sperm bank. While frozen sperm is the industry standard, it is less likely to produce a pregnancy than fresh sperm, assuming that the semen is kept at the proper temperature and insemination occurs soon after ejaculation.[13]

In a typical medical insemination, the doctor provides the semen of an anonymous genitor to a married couple, who will conceal the origins of the offspring. The husband's infertility is hidden, and the resulting children are spared the presumably painful knowledge and stigma of their "unnatural" extramarital origins.[14]

At The Margins of Medical Discourse

Until the late 1980s, physicians rarely inseminated known lesbians. By limiting their clientele to married heterosexual couples with a fair amount of discretionary income, physicians played a numerically small but ideologically loaded role in the social control of procreation, especially in states where only physicians can legally perform AI.[15] In their unique power relationship to AI technology, and as possessors of the knowledge necessary to implement it, physicians, individually and through professional societies and boards, have been able to inveigh significantly on behalf of the nuclear family.

Physicians played a gatekeeper role in determining who was a fit "patient" for AI, and hence what child was better off never being conceived. This role is a familiar one for the medical profession, which has only recently and unevenly begun to be divested of its historically unique power over women's procreative lives (e.g., pregnancy, childbirth, abortion, sterilization, contraception). Scholars and activists have argued that the physician's primary role in AI is to serve as an agent of social control—to enforce social norms, values, and prejudices.[16] This role has been exercised in part through physicians' refusal to inseminate lesbians.

The tendency of doctors to reject lesbians for AI services was documented in a 1988 OTA survey, which found that physicians were more likely to reject AI requests from lesbians than from other stigmatized groups of women (some of whom are also lesbians).[17] Doctors were more likely to accept a woman who was "welfare dependent," had medical risks from pregnancy, was infected with syphilis, gonorrhea, genital herpes, hepatitis, cytomegalovirus (CMV), or chlamydia, had a criminal record, had "less than average intelligence," or had less than a high school diploma, than they were to inseminate a known lesbian.[18] Just over ten years later a study by the CDCP found that 79 percent of U.S. fertility clinics treat unmarried women.[19] While the situation of inseminating lesbians has changed profoundly, as recently as 1999 the majority of lesbians inseminating at a clinic in Connecticut had been turned away by other doctors because they were lesbians.[20]

Since its inception, secrecy has been the accepted medical protocol and near-universal norm for AI. Secrecy enables the married couple to achieve the appearance of conjugal fertility, as well as the nuclear family structure sanctioned by religion, gender prerogatives, and the state. By helping the married couple hide the father's lack of biological paternity, AI helps destigmatize what would in a non-medical context be considered adultery or childbirth out of wedlock. At the same time, doctors' classic insistence that AI be performed only within heterosexual marriage reinforces social norms of marriage and nuclear family that contribute to the stigmatization of lesbian families. In this constellation, AI is contractual, anonymous, and apparently non-threatening to patriarchal prerogatives. Medical protocols built around assumptions of conjugal fertility (which are often backed by law and insurance companies alike) disenfranchise lesbians who seek to build families through insemination. Thus, the medical establishment traditionally has worked to contain AI within the boundaries of the nuclear family.

In most countries and states, the law protects the rights of all players in the typical, secretive use of AI within a married, heterosexual couple. Alabama's statute is typical:

§ 26-17-21. *Artificial insemination*

(a) If, under the supervision of a licensed physician and with the consent of her husband, a wife is inseminated artificially with semen donated by a man not her husband, the husband is treated in law as if he were the natural father of a child thereby conceived. The husband's consent must be in writing and signed by him and his wife. The physician shall certify their signatures and the dates of the insemination, and file the husband's consent with the State Department of Health, where it shall be kept confidential and in a sealed file. However, the physician's failure to do so does not affect the father and child relationship. All papers and records pertaining to the insemination, whether part of the permanent record of a court or of a file held by the supervising physician or elsewhere, are subject to inspection only upon an order of the court for good cause shown. The supervising physician shall not be liable to any person, including the wife, the husband, or a child resulting from an artificial insemination procedure, for the release of any information pertaining to the artificial insemination which occurs through accident, error, omission, inadvertence or the intentional conduct, without malice, of the physician or his agents, servants, or employees.

(b) The donor of semen provided to a licensed physician for use in artificial insemination of a married woman other than the donor's wife is treated in law as if he were not the natural father of a child thereby conceived.

The law treats the husband as the father, whose paternal status shields all family members from intrusion by the sperm donor. The sperm donor is likewise protected from paternity claims through medical protocols emphasizing anonymity and by statute. In fact, eight U.S. states have codes specifically sealing records related to AI.[21] The doctor is also protected from lawsuits that might be brought by inseminated women or their offspring seeking to learn the identity of the donor. In this arrangement, medicine, law, and the nuclear family are nearly seamless. For most of its history, AI fit nicely into the (patriarchal) norms of medicine, family, and law.

A major change in this scenario came in the 1970s, when lesbians and other unmarried women, emboldened by the women's and gay liberation movements, began to inseminate, outside the medical context, with the explicit intention of mothering without men.[22] This shift was to shatter the apparently natural unity of medicine, families, and the law embodied in conventional uses of AI.

Lesbian families reconstruct these norms, creatively negotiating the damning discourses of medical and psychological experts as well as the complex politics of lesbian family resemblance. Lesbians have both demedicalized AI and created new options for medical AI that expose the heterosexist ideology of conventional AI practices.

Lesbians have also generated numerous innovative legal approaches to protecting intentional lesbian families and family members. Some of these legal strategies use conservative patriarchal family tropes. Others challenge assumptions about the normative family. Motherhood historically has had to be constrained within a particular kind of family to be considered "legitimate." Which families are deemed socially and legally legitimate changes across time, place, and culture. Legal marriage, racist and ablist eugenic criteria, middle class status, being sexually monogamous with one's husband, and other criteria are all factors in a matrix of status hierarchies that determine a mother's access to "legitimacy." With lesbian self-insemination, women flout these proscriptions, and claim the traditionally male prerogative of heading a household.[23]

Far from being "just like" coital impregnation, the practice of lesbian AI problematizes some of our most sacred and taken-for-granted assumptions about the family and gender arrangements. Alternative insemination continues the disaggregation of motherhood and fatherhood that the new procreative technologies represent, and separates the sexual and paternal significance of semen from its procreative function. Arguably, this level of disaggregation has moved beyond the differentiation that characterizes modernity into a new realm of (postmodern) disconnection. The intentional lesbian family is a postmodern family form that emphasizes affinity over both biology and (patri)lineage. Sociologist Judith Stacey aptly uses the term "postmodern family" ". . . to signal the contested, ambivalent, and undecided character of our contemporary family cultures."[24]

Political pundits, psychological "experts," policy makers, and other purveyors of conventional wisdom would have us believe that fatherhood is the *sine qua non* of healthy family and child development. This view negates the validity of lesbian families. It was typified by *Bowers v. Hardwick,* in which the United States Supreme Court, in ruling that states may continue to outlaw homosexuality, pronounced: "No connection between family, marriage, or procreation on the one hand and homosexual activity on the other has been demonstrated."[25] Yet the lesbian baby boom shows that each year thousands of mentally and socially well-adjusted children are brought into the world and raised by lesbians, generally in families without fathers.

Despite variations across states and countries, the lesbian baby boom spans the wealthy nations. It has emerged in a context in which both "alternative" families and procreative technologies are increasingly normalized.[26] Developed countries are currently in the midst of

> the modern transformation of marriage from a hierarchical, gender-polarized relationship whose permanence was enforced by God, law, family and community into a more equal, fluid, and optional relationship whose permanence depends on the mutual wishes of the partners.[27]

Intentional lesbian motherhood is a result, not a cause, of the shifting family terrain. This terrain includes the proliferation of technological and contractual procreation since the mid-1980s. In this context, one cannot assume that a child is living with her biological parents or that she was conceived through heterosexual intercourse. Diverse family forms—nonmarital births, divorce, same-sex marriage, non-marital cohabitation, interracial couples, blended families, and double-income couples—have proliferated. Lesbian AI both contributes to, and emerged from, the social and technological conditions of the last quarter of the twentieth century, to create its own brand of baby-making and kinship arrangements. Lesbian AI epitomizes the new, postmodern family.

> Queer families occupy the vanguard of the postmodern family condition, because they make the denaturalized and contingent character of family and kinship impossible to ignore.[28]

Which arrangements of kin will be deemed legitimate? Only those sanctioned by marriage? Only those linked by blood ties? How do the relationships among self-defined families stand up to challenges from those claiming parental rights based on biology, and vice versa? What do the courts have to say about the legitimacy of various family configurations, and how do they justify those decisions? What parental rights does a sperm donor have? Do such rights hinge on the participation of a doctor or the marriage of the mother to a man? What legal rights does a lesbian co-mother have vis-à-vis her (not biologically related) child?

Stacey compares the state's treatment of postmodern families in the United States and in Scandinavia to highlight the punitive nature of the U.S. response to shifting family demographics.[29] Scandinavian countries have responded to increased single motherhood by increasing state subsidies so that few women and children live in poverty. The United States, on the other hand, has severed even some of the most basic welfare state guarantees, and a quarter of U.S. children live in poverty. Stacey tersely comments that:

> There seems to be a nearly inverse relationship between a nation's rhetorical concern over the plight of children in declining families and its willingness to implement policies to ease their suffering . . . Lip service to the family . . . serves as a proxy for the private sphere and as a rationale for abdicating public responsibility for social welfare.[30]

The state (via courts, politicians, laws, and policies) generally locates immorality in the sphere of "deviant" sexuality, and thus deflects attention from its own immorality, its complicity in sexual politics, its racism, its explicit (military, police, penal) violence and its implicit sanction of "private" domestic and economic violence against women, children, and other vulnerable members of society. Morality, as sociologist M. Jacqueline Alexander points out, is always a feminist issue.[31] As long as immorality is deflected from the state onto sexuality, lesbians and their families will be scapegoated, and the state will continue to be immoral.

Medicine, Religion, Law, and Families

Patriarchal institutions operate simultaneously and synergistically to support patriarchal power. Medical and legal discourses around AI work together to support the normative—though far from numerically predominant—heteropatriarchal family and to shore up its dominance at the expense of other kinship arrangements. These discourses are not seamless, however, but contain internal contradictions that "outsiders" have exploited to gain rights and freedoms.

Medicine has one set of practices and discourses around AI, which prop up certain ideological stories about "The Family." The law tells its own stories, as well as being the arena where struggles over legitimacy and rights for non-nuclear families get hashed out. Lesbians tell another story. These (differently) powerful discourses mark the terrain in which lesbians fight for their right to create, live, and define their families the way they see fit.

Both medicine and the law have long institutional histories, variously intertwined with state power. Legal scholar Mary Eaton notes that "law can be reconceptualized . . . as productive and not simply repressive, and the legal can therefore be conceived as a sphere in which identity is constituted rather than reflected."[32] Medicine, too, generates and manages subjectivities[33]; medicine not only disciplines our bodies and minds, but shapes them deeply. Both law and medicine can be instruments of oppression as well as life-saving protection. Both also wield massive moral authority to declare people "sick" or "healthy," "guilty" or "innocent," morally and physiologically "wrong" or "right."

The practices of AI are regulated in a number of ways both within the United States and around the world. New Zealand political scientist

Robert Blank succinctly locates the forms of AI regulation on a continuum from lesser to greater regulation:

1. Individual physicians;
2. Program guidelines;
3. Professional association guidelines;
4. Commissions, committees, task forces;
5. Government guidelines;
6. Licensing regulations;
7. Legislation.[34]

It is clear from looking at this list that the medical and legal systems work in tandem to regulate the practice of AI. While the softest form of regulation in the above list is medical and the hardest is legal, regulation does not progress linearly from the medical to legal. Rather, both sources of regulation have their softer and harder modes.

Defenders of "traditional family values" often feel directly challenged by the existence of lesbian AI. Depending on the time and place, lesbian families and family members may be outlawed, condemned, damned, or, in rare cases, tolerated. Male-dominated societies typically look to religion (along with law, medicine, and custom) to justify male supremacy. The extent to which the tautology of male god/male supremacy/father right is still held sacred in modern societies is often veiled, however, until a family's boundaries transgress the status quo. Father-right may be encoded in legal, medical, and/or religious texts, and may operate consciously and/or unconsciously, but those who violate it feel the repercussions. As poet and essayist Adrienne Rich writes,

> "Father-right" must be seen as one specific form of the rights men are presumed to enjoy simply because of their gender: the "right" to the priority of male over female needs, to sexual and emotional services from women, to women's undivided attention in any and all situations.[35]

The sexual politics of lesbian families (and in some countries the cultural politics of procreative technologies) are so antithetical to male dominance that not only religious authorities, but also secular governments, have felt the need to publicly condemn lesbians, reproductive technology, same-sex marriage, and/or lesbian AI.

Boom

While the lesbian baby boom is widely perceived as a phenomenon that began in the 1980s, the University of Wisconsin study reported that, as early as 1977, 9.5 percent of the doctors surveyed had been approached by an unmarried woman (some of whom we may assume were lesbians) for insemination services.[36] The earliest printed reference I have been able to find to lesbian insemination is a listing for a workshop offered as part of the 1975 Conference on Women and Health at the Harvard Medical School. The workshop, offered by Helen Donaldson, was called "Lesbians: Artificial Insemination at Home."[37] Doubtless, lesbians were inseminating before this conference took place.

These new lesbian practices of AI were and are as diverse as lesbians themselves. Some lesbians prefer the privacy, legal security, and/or greater control of the child's health provided by choosing an anonymous sperm donor from a semen bank. Others welcome the chance to have a known sperm donor with whom their child can have a relationship of some kind, or at least the possibility of contact when the child grows up. In one study, 57 percent of lesbians and single heterosexual women who undertook AI said they would like their child-to-be to be able to meet the sperm donor.[38] Some mothers-to-be prefer what they perceive as greater control of the health and genetic traits conferred by medically screened semen. Others prefer to enlist a trusted male friend or family member of the non-inseminating partner to provide sperm, even if he may not have a perfect health history. Some lesbians prefer to have the insemination performed by a doctor so that intra-uterine insemination can be used, enabling costs to be covered by insurance, or simply because it feels more comfortable to them. Others gain a greater feeling of autonomy, control, and comfort by inseminating at home, perhaps with the help of a friend or partner. Such diverse practices of AI, as well as lesbians intentionally becoming parents in other ways (e.g., adoption, foster parenting, or co-parenting a partner's child) have fueled the lesbian baby boom. This baby boom has involved thousands of lesbians engaging in complex negotiations of maternal and lesbian identities and social networks, as well as considerable ingenuity in non-patriarchal family- and baby- making.[39] Lesbians have built, and continue to build, counter-discourses and counter-institutions to support their families and to help them negotiate the powerful heterosexist institutions they must deal with as lesbians and as mothers.

Discerning the dimensions of the lesbian baby boom, or the number of children born through lesbian AI, is impossible since we have few hard numbers to work with. Compounding the difficulties of quantifying an unregulated, out-of-hospital "medical" procedure is the intractable problem of counting "homosexuals." University of Michigan law professor David L. Chambers writes:

> In one effort to survey Americans in every state by phone, it took 1,650 calls to Kansas—55 hours of random dialing—before the pollsters found the first person willing to admit being lesbian or gay . . . It is possible of course that fewer than one tenth of one percent of Kansans are gay, but I doubt it.[40]

This problem grows exponentially when trying to determine the number of lesbian mothers, who are often even more vulnerable to homophobia than those without children. Undaunted by the lack of hard data, I contend that the lesbian baby boom is in fact booming.

Physician and lesbian health activist Kate O'Hanlan performed a thorough review of the international data on the incidence of lesbianism from countries including Japan, Thailand, Denmark, France, the Republic of Palau, Great Britain, and Australia. Her review found that 0.2 to 6.9 percent of women describe themselves as lesbians.

> The surveys reviewed suggest that of the sixty-five million women in the United States, 3.6% are lesbians. This means that our country is home to some 2.3 million lesbian citizens. Over 69,000 lesbian couples identified themselves in the 1990 census count, which is an unknown fraction of the lesbian population.[41]

She adds that no study of lesbians has ever validated the popularly quoted figure that 10 percent of women are lesbians.

We also lack data to determine how many inseminations are performed in the United States. Lesbian AI has grown and changed tremendously since the last time data on AI was collected in 1987. In that year, 6 percent of U.S. women seeking AI reported to their physicians that they were unmarried, and an additional 1 percent did not disclose marital status. Of the unmarried 6 percent, 2 percent reported living in a couple with a man, 3 percent reported being heterosexual and single, and 1 percent reported being in a lesbian couple.[42]

If we take these figures at face value, they translate into around 4,000 requests from single women and 1,000 requests from lesbians during a one-year period.[43] I do not think it is wise, however, to take these figures at face value, since a realistic fear of discrimination leads many lesbians to claim to be heterosexual in order to receive medical services. Even if we eliminate the approximately 3,000 women who report cohabiting with a man and the approximately 4,000 who report being heterosexual and single, we arrive at a significant pool of inseminating women who may in fact be lesbian (some of the married women may be lesbians as well). When the lesbians who self-inseminated outside of the medical system are added, the possible number of inseminating lesbians skyrockets, since these numbers were collected at a time when most physicians denied insemination services to known lesbians.[44]

Despite a shortage of hard numbers, evidence of the lesbian baby boom abounds. In laws and other legal documents, we find legislation and legal rulings regulating lesbian insemination and parenting. We find further proof of the prevalence of lesbian AI practices in domestic and international position papers written by both medical and human rights bodies. We can see lesbian family contingents in gay pride marches, as well as lesbian-parent families in neighborhoods, schools, and parks. We can survey books, papers, articles, internet sites, listservs, and other publications about lesbian-parent families. Finally, we can look at the large (in)fertility industry that offers (and withholds) services to lesbians. While such oblique evidence does not render hard numbers, it does affirm the perception that lesbian AI is a robust and widespread phenomenon.

Methodologies

Lesbian AI is surprisingly undertheorized, particularly when compared to the voluminous work published each year on other forms of technological and contractual procreation. Lesbian AI has been included in discussions of other, related social phenomena, but rarely as a distinct issue.

Discussions of lesbian and gay parenting rarely analyze the sexism that underlies much discrimination suffered by lesbians.[45] Discussions of the legal situations of lesbian, gay, bisexual, and transgender (LGBT) people suffer from a tendency to de-emphasize important differences between lesbians and gay men.[46] Discussions of lesbian parenting generally include AI as one of the many practical, technical, political, and theoretical issues relevant to lesbian mothers.[47] But these considerations tend to focus on the practicalities of achieving pregnancy and/or the role of the sperm donor.

Alternative insemination gets limited attention in debates about contractual and technological procreation since the main focus is usually the more intrusive forms of reproductive technology.[48] Discussions of having babies without men that are geared toward heterosexual women do not emphasize lesbian realities.[49] Lastly, a single book addresses social science approaches to AI, and it does not center on lesbians.[50]

While lesbian AI overlaps with these and other subjects, theorizing lesbian AI is limited when it is seen merely as an adjunct topic to the "real" matter at hand. Scholars, artists, and activists from a host of disciplines have shown that "shifting the center" is a transformative process rather than just an additive one.[51] Accordingly, focusing on lesbian AI uniquely illuminates the family, gender, and cultural norms that are invisible when no such shift occurs. While it cannot be theorized in isolation from other important social realities, such as race, class, and nationality, we still lack an expansive delineation of the issues and stakes raised by lesbian AI. My hope here is to begin walking that road.

2

Setting the Historical Stage

ABSTRACT

Social control in modernity is achieved in large part by policing the body, with special reference to its origins and privileges as indicated by parentage (e.g., sperm, blood, and name). The family, in its aspect as an extension of the state, has been an important locus of social control under the guise of the natural. As lesbian AI uncouples and demystifies sperm, sexuality, and kinship, it threatens to throw that entire set of delineators out the window. At the same time, the commercialization of the sperm used in lesbian AI is fraught with paradoxes and contradictions. What I have done here is assemble an admittedly idiosyncratic history of issues relevant to lesbian AI. I discuss early insemination practices and changes in the medical profession's openness to lesbian AI. I focus on changing views of sperm in order to map shifts in racially and sexually stratified family norms. I also explore historical changes in the structure of families, the social role of sperm, eugenic implications of sperm banking, and lesbians as "bad mothers." This discussion sets the stage for understanding how lesbian inseminators both transgress the intended (heteronormative and eugenic) uses of AI and become high-paying accomplices.

Premodern, Modern, and Ultramodern Family Structures

The basic form of European and American families has shifted over the past three hundred years or so. Roughly speaking, we began with the pre-modern (or "feudal") family, which is patriarchal and naturalistic.

Then we moved to the modern family, which is contractarian and characterized by more equality and autonomy among members. Finally we arrived at the ultramodern ("postmodern") family, which I will describe in more depth. While we can map the transformations of families from the more feudal to the more modern in various settings, there has not been an unambiguous "evolution" in which an oppressive family has given way to an egalitarian one. Neither has there been simply a collapse, by which what was good and wholesome in the family has been replaced by loveless and Godless atomization. No clean break demarcated the hegemony of pre-modern and modern family forms. Rather, feudal (overtly patriarchal) and modern (capitalist) conceptions of the family have areas of congruence and conflict with each other.

My use of the terms pre-modern, modern, and postmodern is not intended to suggest that these are discrete and "real" entities. I have yet to be convinced that our contemporary period is "post-" modernity. Neither have I been persuaded that feudal Europe was "pre-" modern in the etiological sense of inevitable stages that constitute Eurocentric ideologies of progress. And there is no such thing, empirically, as "the (singular) modern family." Rather, there have been many types of household and kinship arrangements within each period. Contingent and hybrid social forms, including households and kinship groups, have always existed and co-existed with more (stereo)typically feudal and modern ones.[1] Having made that disclaimer, I use the terms "pre-modern," "modern," and "postmodern" in order to write more clearly about the meanings and politics of AI among lesbians.[2]

I offer here a brief chronology of some of the major developments in kinship arrangements that most directly affect and frame the current situation of lesbian AI. I begin this (broadly drawn) sketch in feudal Europe, before the industrial revolution, when, for the vast majority of men, women, and children, family and work had no functional separation. In these pre-modern, precapitalist economies, the household was overtly patriarchal and patrilineal. The father was the legal ruler, if not owner, of the other members of the family. His name, land, and other property, if any, were passed on to his male heirs. In this context, childbearing followed the "flowerpot model" of pregnancy.[3] As early as classical times, a man's "seed" was alleged to contain what would become the child, which temporarily roomed in its mother's body, until it could be born.[4] Plato, for instance, believed that women's sole contribution to procreation was their menstrual blood. In the words of feminist philosopher Mary O'Brien,

> [The] idea that women contribute only "material" to babies while men contribute spirit or soul or some other human "essence" must have struck chords in the masculine imagination, for it lingered for centuries.[5]

In all versions of this view, children were understood as children of their fathers, the children of men. Girls and women married exogamously, and would give up their fathers' name and take on that of their husbands. In the rare event that parents divorced, the man got custody of the children, who were considered his property. At this time, the home was not especially associated with women, nor was there a separate sphere of "work" that was the domain of men. The pre-modern family was underpinned by ideologies of nature and the natural, with the family itself, as well as the roles within it, understood as "natural" and "right."

In feudal Europe, power was patriarchal, extremely hierarchical and grounded in metaphors of nature. In the church, the state, and the family, those on top dominated those below, with a rationale based in God's nature. The heteropatriarchal family was seen as natural and Godly; the subordination of women in the church was seen as sacred and "natural." The state enforced its will through a law that was determined "from above" by men who inherited their power in lines of succession and rules of inheritance that were both divinely decided and natural.

The advent of industrialism and the growth of capitalism initiated widespread changes in kinship arrangements. During this process, two distinct spheres, one public and one private, came to be delineated, which were marked by gender. Work moved from the home to the factory, and the home's focus changed from production to procreation, nurturing, domesticity, and use value. In modernity, power remained hierarchical, but was organized ostensibly along more contractarian lines. It is worth considering the proposition that in this Euro-American turn from feudal to modern societies, the patriarchal rule of the fathers has shifted into a fraternistic, although still phallic, regime of the brother.[6] In modernity, the state became democratic, the Protestant Reformation aimed to reduce the power of the church hierarchy (as did *le mort de Dieu*), and the family became increasingly seen as a voluntary contract.

Following World War II, a second dramatic shift in U.S. household and kinship structure unfolded. Postwar affluence precipitated the transformation of the United States from a producer to a consumer society. This change arguably contributed to a dramatic transformation in male role expectations in order that men could become the kind of consumers that the postwar conditions of capital necessitated. Judith Stacey writes that the "postmodern family" signifies

> the contested, ambivalent, and undecided character of our contemporary family cultures . . . Like postmodern culture, contemporary Western family arrangements are diverse, fluid, and unresolved. Like postmodern cultural forms, our families today admix unlikely elements in an improvisational pastiche of old and new.[7]

Disrupting the seemingly "logical" historical progression from feudal to modern family forms, the postmodern family condition reflects postmodern economic, cultural, and political conditions in which (to quote Yeats) "the center does not hold." As Stacey says,

> The postmodern family condition is not a new model of family life equivalent to that of the modern family; it is not the next stage in an orderly progression of stages of family history; rather the postmodern family condition signals the moment in that history when our belief in a logical progression of stages has broken down. . . . [T]he postmodern family condition incorporates both experimental and nostalgic dimensions as it lurches forward and backward into an uncertain future.[8]

The center of the postmodern family splits apart in many ways. Today, for example, resources are still controlled unequally by those in power, but both the law and God's nature have lost much of their power as foundational metaphors. Anthropologist Susan Martha Kahn describes this shift, drawing on the insights of fellow anthropologists Sarah Franklin and Marilyn Strathern:

> The new reproductive technologies and the Euro-American "enterprise" culture in which they are deployed have turned nature into an anachronism; it no longer exists as an idiom unto itself but has become

context-dependent. Once it was the context, it was the field from which metaphor emerged; now nature has simply become flattened into a market concept that depends on the consumer's invocation of it in order to come into being. This conceptual shift is profoundly destabilizing to Euro-American beliefs about kinship, where kinship has been understood as a fact of society rooted in facts of nature, or as that which connects the domains of nature and culture.[9]

In Euro-American metaphysics, nature once was the source of metaphors. Now market values have reduced nature to one metaphor among many. This shift transforms the way that Euro-Americans see themselves.[10] Where once they were products of (God's) nature, now they are products of (parents') consumer choices.

Semen Donors, Paternity, and Patriarchy

In a similar shift, the law of the land still holds a great deal of power, but state power and patriarchal power are exercised through a wide range of social institutions and discourses. Foucault writes,

> I do not mean to say that the law fades into the background or that the institutions of justice tend to disappear, but rather that the law operates more and more as a norm, and that the judicial institution is increasingly incorporated into a continuum of apparatuses (medical, administrative, and so on) whose functions are for the most part regulatory.[11]

Sperm donors exercise both the biological and the social freedoms enabled by paternity under patriarchy. Men's biological freedom from reproductive labor (pregnancy, childbirth, lactation) enables sperm donors, like all biological fathers, to have "something (reproduction) for [almost] nothing (ejaculation)."[12] At the same time, male-made legal traditions provide the legal freedom to claim or disavow social paternity.

Feudal patrilineage translated rather neatly into a modern family system ("capitalist-patriarchy"). While this family form's hegemony is hardly guaranteed, its grounding in private property and accumulation kept it a fairly cohesive "marriage."[13] Capitalist-patriarchy is an analytic category developed by socialist feminists trying to understand the structures of domination in their lives and in the world.[14] While the term capitalist-patriarchy was coined in the early 1970s, socialist feminists have for more than a hundred years worked to integrate across the hyphen, struggling against the reduction of either term to a function of the other.[15] In this approach, which strongly influences my work, it is impossible to analyze either capitalism or patriarchy without analyzing the other.[16] On the other hand, ideas about sperm are an area where the two kinship models diverge and come into open conflict: Today we find representations of (feudal) sperm-as-sacred-seed-of-life and (modern) sperm-as-commodity.[17]

Societies, individuals, religions, and professions have distinctive views of sperm, which are connected to larger cultural narratives regarding reproduction, bodies and sexuality, manhood and womanhood, fatherhood and motherhood. These views strongly influence how groups and individuals conceptualize and react to the prospect of AI. Interwoven with various understandings of women's place in the family and the world, and women's sexuality, views about semen shape how insemination is viewed, organized, and regulated.

Some authors compare semen providers to those who relinquish children for adoption. They argue that in AI, the biological fathers relinquish their parental rights and responsibilities before their children even exist, before, in fact, conception even occurs. They point out that this is allowed in many states under a different set of rules than governs the relinquishment of actual children, since all states require a waiting period after a child is born during which the biological mother (and biological father, if he is known) have the right to change their minds. Such adoption laws work on the assumption that the experience of being a parent of a baby is different from the merely intellectual knowledge that one will soon have that baby, and that for some parents that experience is transformative enough to make them decide to keep their child. Some argue that sperm donors should be entitled to this waiting period as well.

Others compare semen providers to blood or bone marrow donors: They contribute a biological substance that their bodies will replenish, at little or no medical risk to themselves. In this view there should be no restrictions on sperm donors except for those necessary for the recipient's, the provider's, and the public's health.

Still others suggest that sperm donors are better compared to vital organ donors, since they give a precious part of themselves that is needed by others to save (or, in the case of AI, create) a life. In this view, sperm donors should be socially acknowledged as generous donors who play a vital role in the lives of others. Whether they are rewarded financially would hinge on ethical questions about how that payment would affect the social relationships among providers, recipients, and their communities. Further, if the sperm donor is someone who "gives the gift of life," he is likely to be seen as someone important in the lives of inseminees and offspring alike.

Some see sperm donors in commercial terms, as producers and merchants of a commodity that has value in the market. In this view, there is no need for sperm donors to consider the results of their contributions, or for physicians to investigate the personhood, feelings, or role of the provider. Instead, the sperm is the focus, and the sperm donor is a means to an end. In the biomedical view, sperm, which can be either commercialized or donated, is a medical "product." It is the basis for the treatment of a disease (infertility), and needs to be obtained and processed in the safest, most effective way possible to best treat the patient. The sperm donor disappears into the background as soon as his sperm is obtained, except inasmuch as tracking him is necessary to the future health of the recipient and offspring.

Sperm as Commodity

Donated sperm can be viewed as both manifestation and agent of social stratification. Semen is sorted and classified according to hierarchical categories of social and physical dominance. Qualities believed to signal "good genes" such as race, education, sexual orientation, strength, height, robust health, attractiveness, professional success, and talent in areas such as math, music, and athletics are carefully identified. The "value" of sperm is based on the provider's social location vis-à-vis various axes of social privilege and power.

Finally, from an entrepreneurial perspective, sperm is a product that can be profitably enhanced and marketed.

> [Sperm banks] can increase demand in the semen market by convincing or, better yet, guaranteeing the general public that technosemen is fertile, uncontaminated, and genetically "engineered" for desirable traits. In the age of the AIDS epidemic, geneticism, and increased environ-

mental disasters, semen banks can capitalize on the promise these technological procedures offer . . .[18]

This latter social reality may well be the one that most strongly shapes the practices of contemporary lesbian insemination.

Semen, as the symbol of male "potency," is valorized in patriarchal cultures around the world. Patriarchal religions speak of a man's seed as sacred, precious, not to be "spilled." Semen is valorized in the law, through patrilineage, which defines "fatherhood" in large part as an ejaculatory relationship of genitor to offspring. The fact that buyers, including lesbian buyers, of semen believe such characteristics as college education and "health" to be transmissible through a man's semen is further evidence of the magical thinking about semen that abounds in our culture. It also shows that lesbians are not exempt from such magical thinking or the eugenic and patriarchal discourses that underlie it.

In modernity, sperm is demystified as part of the larger disenchantment of the lifeworld.[19] We move from a naturalistic worldview that imbues things with mystical, traditional and religious collective significance to a world that is rationalized and disenchanted. In postmodernity, re-enchantment is simulated telelectronically and through the fetishization of commodities. This is not a linear process that happens everywhere at the same time and in one direction. Rather, some parts of life resist disenchantment and are especially susceptible to simulated re-enchantment. Procreation is certainly one of them.

With the acceleration of capital in ultramodernity, the commodification of every possible aspect of life, including that which was formerly considered most private and sacred, has intensified. The term "commodification" comes from Marxist analysis that decries the alienation inherent in reducing everything in life to a monetary value. Yet commodification need not only sound an alarm. Turning objects, relationships, people, and ideas into items of sale becomes a fascinating process when we analyze the commercialization of sperm.

Whereas in feudal Europe the monarchy itself hinged on the tight control of gametes among royals, in modernized kinship arrangements the biogenetic tie is still valorized, but less so than in the feudal, and it is also subject to negotiation. This semiotic conflict is epitomized in the transformation of straight-white sperm into commodity. From its feudal status as symbol and agent of male power over women and children (and at times over slaves of all sexes and ages), as well as of class position vis-à-vis inheritance and the family name, white male semen has come a long way into the über-sperm banks of today.

The practice of AI has grown out of and contributed to this transformation. This transformation of the uses of semen was resisted at first, with alarmist feudal family discourse, and accused of marking the downfall of the (patriarchal) family, God, and nation. Controversy raged in the 1950s over the newly publicized practice of AI in the medical community, in the press, and in the British Parliament (where one Lord branded it "a brain wave of Beelzebub"[20]). In fact, the existence of AI was so disturbing to the powers that be on both sides of the Atlantic that legislative bodies in the United States and throughout Western Europe took up the issue, holding commissions and issuing reports about the threats AI posed to the sanctity of life, marriage, and hence God and country.

In 1959, the British House of Lords set up the Feversham Committee to investigate the legal implications of AI. Historian Naomi Pfeffer explains,

> The social issue articulated in the context of the debate about artificial insemination using donor semen in the 1950s was the question of legitimacy. . . . Children conceived through donor semen represented a conscious effort to bring forth an illegitimate child within marriage. Recourse to artificial insemination using donor semen thereby constituted a very subversive act and a direct challenge to the family.[21]

Such sentiments may seem antiquated in this era of cloning and embryos on ice, but they are far from extinct. Legal scholar Holly Harlow details the impediments that such alarmist paternalism still poses to "single women," including lesbians, who seek to inseminate. The harm is particularly direct when physicians hold such beliefs:

> Unfortunately, some physicians ignore the statistics and studies concerning the positive effects of single motherhood on children and maintain discriminatory policies against AID [artificial insemination by donor] of single women because they are influenced by the irrational and inflammatory opinions of some authors.[22]

Harlow goes on to quote "family values" activist David Blankenhorn, who condemns the use of AI by all unmarried women (including lesbians).

> For the culture, the rise of the Sperm Father constitutes nothing less than father killing, the willing enactment of cultural patricide. For the individual man, being a sperm father is not a style of fatherhood but a means of paternal suicide: the collaboration of the male in the eradication of his fatherhood. Toward the end of the fatherless society, the Sperm Father represents the final solution.[23]

Blankenhorn, in his popular book *Fatherless America: Confronting Our Most Urgent Social Problem,* laments what he sees as the demise of fatherhood in America. One of its most reviled aspects is "the Sperm Father," a category that includes all men whose only link to their offspring is sperm—rapists, one-night stands, anonymous sperm donors, helpful male friends, and other moral monsters.[24] Blankenhorn finds horror in the prospect of women opting to inseminate and raise children out of wedlock. He draws on Locke and Hobbes to argue that fatherhood is the barrier between civilization and barbarism. He even threatens a Hobbesian vision of chaos if we fail to retreat from the moral precipice represented by the insemination of unmarried women.

> Today's reemergence of the Sperm Father as a mass male phenomenon constitutes our society's clearest example of cultural regression. In political philosophy terms, the Sperm Father signifies a relapse from society to the state of nature.[25]

In other words, the existence of insemination outside of heterosexual marriage is not merely personally revolting to Blankenhorn. Rather, it presages an apocalyptic "return" to an imagined pre patriarchal past fraught with brutality, chaos, and aggression. Blankenhorn draws on John Locke's seventeenth-century fantasy of male sexual behavior in "the state of nature" before patriarchy.

> Here is male sexuality freed from societal norms. It is asocial copulation, impersonal impregnation. It is frequently predatory and violent. Call it unenculturated male procreation: fatherhood in the state of nature. It is the original model of the Sperm Father.[26]

This portrayal is profoundly shaped by colonial myths of "savage" sexuality and the civilizing power of Europe, here cast as the civilizing power of biolegal paternity.

Conservative "family values" authors such as Blankenhorn seem almost parodic in their doom-saying about insemination. From the Tories of nineteenth-century England to the "pro-family" pundits of the present, we can see that the specter of autonomous motherhood (and demystified sperm) strikes fear into the hearts of phallic pundits.

The commodification of semen also places the practice of AI near the limits of legal contract. While it is still illegal, technically, to sell sexual acts, body parts, and babies, the seemingly infinite reach of capitalism ensures that the boundaries of these prohibitions will continue to be pushed.[27] Semen itself—determinant of social class status, signifier of father right, and/or technologically mediated commodity—is an example *prima facie*. Certainly AI commodifies a substance (semen) long considered "priceless" if not sacred, and inseparable from sexual and paternal significance.

In our ultracapitalist economy, modernization advances to the point that even bodily products and processes are monetarily valuated and exchanged on the "free market." Blood, organs, sex, and childcare are for sale, wombs are for rent, and a variety of semen "flavors" are available for a price from the sperm bank. It was in this postwar ultramodern social economy that AI became widely available. As sociologist Dion Farquhar writes,

> Reproductive technologies . . . are the legacy of post–World War II advances in agribusiness such as animal husbandry breeding techniques and animal medical research . . . Other, allied technologies such as fiber optics, ultrasound, laser diagnostics and surgery, and microsurgery are inextricable from their original military weapons associations and later commercial applications . . . [and] from the context of its development by international corporate capital, from the degree and kind of state support it receives, and from its differential national reception and distribution . . .[28]

These "advances" in technoscience are inextricable from the growth of lesbian AI and its integration into flows of liquid capital.[29]

With the help of modernist medical discourses, however, AI has become widely acceptable and recuperable into the parameters of the nuclear family. As a "treatment" for the married, heterosexual, white, middle-class, "tragic" subfertile couple, AI became sufficiently non-threatening that public opinion—as reflected in and shaped by the press, legislature, and later, public opinion polls—found AI to be, if not dinner-time conversation, at least rescued from narratives of animal husbandry and deemed securely "civilized."[30] It was determined that as long as AI served to enhance the law-abiding nuclear family, under the watchful eye of medical authorities, it was probably an upright treatment after all. Safely nuclearized and medicalized, a limited form of AI became acceptable even to the Pope—just as long as the semen derived from the lawfully wedded husband of the woman who was being inseminated.[31] Even among heterosexuals, however, AI is not actually a treatment for male infertility. It is a procedure performed on women with no impact on a male partner's fertility.[32]

"Blood," Sperm, and Human Engineering

The meanings of "blood," (which commingle with the meanings of sperm) are similarly contested in postmodern times. One's "blood" was all-determining of one's conditions in life under feudalism and only somewhat less so as Europe and its colonies modernized. But in capitalist economies, we see the rise of ideologies of opportunity, self-made men, and meritocracy, which reflect changing class structures that demand modernist discourses (rather than those of "blood") for legitimation. At the same time, such individualist discourses mask the persistence of "blood" as a major determinant of one's "station" in life.

O'Brien suggests that Plato's particular "flowerpot model" of pregnancy, in which women are believed to contribute nothing but menstrual blood to procreation, may have been widely held in antiquity and may have contributed to the linguistic development that understands kin as blood relations.[33] It is important to remember that "blood" (race, family name and property, maleness and femaleness) is never just blood. Biogenetic (blood) ties are powerful symbolic signifiers for what we ingrain deeply by coding as "natural." "The natural" itself is in no way reducible to those meanings attributed to it in Western signifying systems. Nature is not necessarily stable, eternal, normal, physiological, cultural, feminine, dumb, unchangeable, inert, pure, authentic, or inanimate. But our linking of terms and concepts such as "blood" and "natural" is significant.

At a level only sometimes below the conscious, lesbian AI evokes pre-existing Western discourses around dangerous sexuality, tainted blood (lines), and degeneracy, all threats to family and state.[34] The concept of blood has long been used in Western history to denigrate and oppress others. These discourses have been deployed not only against inseminating lesbians, but also against gay men, colonized people and their descendants, "foreigners," illegal drug users, and prostitutes.[35] Blood is a code word for race, with connotations regarding the sanctity of blood, mixing blood, white blood, black blood, and pure versus tainted blood. Chattel slavery was legitimized in part by maintaining rigid boundaries between the races with morally-biologically calculated categories such as white and black blood. Today, Native Americans are still granted or denied recognition by the United States government based on "blood quantum." In racist cultures such as that of the United States, "non-whites" are identified by their blood, always in opposition to the ostensibly "pure blooded" "white" person.

The theory of degeneracy—evolution in reverse—deserves mention, as it continues to haunt our thinking about reproduction, race, and "normality." The theory of degeneracy, highly influential in nineteenth- and twentieth-century Western sciences, was based on the belief in "evolutionary" progress from genetically inferior to genetically superior organisms (including human beings), which was believed to be the foundation of social "progress." Social and biological progress was understood in class and racial terms, with white males of the owning class at the top of the evolutionary heap.

This progress, however, was always threatened by "degeneracy," which would reverse not only social but biological progress. This threat was embodied by people whom scientists deemed "degenerate." Depending on the time, place, and scientific expert, this group included non-"whites," poor people, criminals, the "feeble minded," the insane, "savages," immigrants, people with disabilities, prostitutes, Jews, communists, cross-dressers, syphilitics, and "perverts" of all stripes—the latter group explicitly including lesbians.[36] As independent scholar Martha Gibson points out, the list of categories of people who were labeled degenerates is "long and intertwined." She further notes:

> The web of associations and mutual links that surrounded female homosexual activity and other marginal social groups a century ago lend a perspective to many current issues facing lesbians, gay men, people of color, poor people, women, and other groups that are condemned by the most powerful members of American society.[37]

All these issues come into play with AI—where, along with homophobia, we encounter hemophobia: a fear of blood out of control.[38] German historian Klaus Theweleit argues that anxieties regarding the loss of father right, in which men are in legal and physical control of "their" blood (family), are intolerable under phallic symbolic regimes. The mixing of stranger and kin, and the introduction of extralegal blood (semen) into the womb in AI is intolerable to the rigid ego structures of patriarchal males.[39] When the woman is a "degenerate" (literally: genetically defective) lesbian, it only heightens the grotesquery.

The concept of degeneracy has long been linked to the practice of eugenics. The history of eugenics—the use of medical power to shape the genetic makeup of the human race—includes both "positive" and "negative" practices. Eugenics not only denies procreative options to certain "classes" of people, in this case lesbians, but includes both positive eugenics to encourage "good" births, and negative eugenics to prevent "unfit" births. The basic premise of eugenics, the improvement of the human race through control of breeding, apparently retains an enduring appeal, as well as an enduring aura of horror. While we like to think of Nazi eugenics as a discrete historical phenomenon, eugenics exists along a continuum, with the systematic murder of Jews, homosexuals, people with disabilities, and other "degenerate" undesirables marking an extreme. On the other end of the continuum, we find innocuous or even benign practices such as voluntary, individual screening for serious genetic diseases. Along the continuum, we have more and less gray areas, as well as slippery slopes.

The medical profession continues to be ambivalent about its role in human engineering. In a situation such as AI where the physician can directly affect the creation of a new life, eugenic tendencies often come to the fore. Physicians' reluctance to inseminate lesbians can be seen at least in part as the desire to prevent the birth of more ("genetically flawed") homosexuals. The fact that lesbianism is a socially constructed category, not a genetic one, has not dissuaded those, including lesbians, who believe it to be genetically determined.

Unfortunately, dealing with sperm banks throws lesbians back into the standard ideology of fitness, normality, and desirability, as the selection of semen is fraught with eugenic assumptions. The typical list of sperm donors at a sperm bank reads like a menu at a eugenics restaurant.[40]

The eugenic implications of AI and other procreative technologies can hardly be avoided. In the sperm bank catalogues, for instance, "fair" skinned Caucasians are heavily represented, as are those with higher education, since sperm banks typically recruit sperm donors from local universities. Certainly the anecdotal evidence is that clients of all persuasions generally express interest in sperm donors who are tall, not "fat" or "stocky," formally educated, "fair," and with high incomes. For instance, in one U.S. study, the lesbians and single heterosexual women polled placed the highest value on the sperm donor's education, ethnicity, and height.[41] None of these preferences are geared simply toward optimizing their future children's health.

On-line donor catalogues enable shoppers to select from a dizzying array of donor characteristics. One can search for semen from donors by characteristics such as racial group, height, weight, hair color and texture, eye color, and blood type. One can seek donors of a particular religion, from "Agnostic" to "Sikh," by nationality from "Afghani" to "Yugoslavian," and by occupation from "Accounting" to "Sociology."[42]

The client is sometimes offered the option of purchasing "sex-preselected" semen for an additional fee. However, the American Society for Reproductive Medicine (ASRM), in a report on sex preselection, asserts that there is no proven way to increase the likelihood of producing a boy or a girl before insemination.[43] Despite a "lack of demonstrated efficacy," they lament, "some centers in the United States have continued to use [various] methods, basing their projections of success on highly questionable data that could mislead patients."

One example of this false advertising comes from a U.S. sperm bank, which makes the following claim for its patented method of sex pre-selection:

> Currently, MicroSort sperm separation for female gender selection (XSort) results in an average of 88% X-bearing sperm in the sorted specimen. MicroSort sperm separation for male gender selection (YSort) currently results in an average of 73% Y-bearing sperm in the sorted specimen.[44]

The implication is that sex-preselection will be 88 percent effective for girls and 73 percent effective for boys. Although this method is still in clinical trials, and therefore experimental, its cost starts at $2,550 and rises rapidly.

Another U.S. sperm bank offers "sex selection" for male offspring only.

> Male sex selection is performed on fresh semen using the Ericsson Method (Gametrics Limited). It should be noted that while this method may increase the chances of conceiving a male offspring, results are not guaranteed.[45]

This bank goes on to note that sex selection will add $475 to the cost of insemination on Monday through Saturday, and $685 on Sundays and holidays. (This is a retreat from the same sperm bank's 1991 statement that "results to date indicate 80% reliability for *male* selection and 65% reliability for *female* selection"[46]). Sadly, there is enough of a market for choosing the sex of one's baby-to-be that sperm banks frequently offer sex-preselection to their customers.

In the United States, the development of semen banking is embroiled in eugenic efforts to improve the human race. The banking of "superior" semen, particularly that of "geniuses" such as Nobel Prize winners, was the motivation of the first semen banks, including the infamous Repository for Germinal Choice (better known as the Nobel Prize Sperm Bank) in Encenito, California, that offered sperm it believed would "improve the human gene pool."[47] An entire body of frightening literature documents the eugenic underpinnings of genetics as a scientific discipline in general, and semen banking in particular.[48]

Racial divisions are strictly enforced in semen banking, sometimes to the point of parody. The same sperm bank described above uses a complicated race-based labeling system designed to ensure that the buyer(s) get what they paid for. As the instructional-promotional materials explain,

COLOR-CODING TO DISTINGUISH THE RACIAL
GROUP OF A DONOR
A WHITE cap and WHITE cane indicate a CAUCASIAN donor.
A BLACK cap and BLACK cane indicate a BLACK donor.
A YELLOW cap and YELLOW cane indicate an ASIAN donor.
A RED cap and RED cane indicate ALL OTHER donors.
The ALL OTHER category includes donors with the following ancestries: East Indian, American Indian, Mexican, Latin American,
South and Central American, Samoan, Hawaiian, Pacific Islander,
and donors with mixed racial background.

IMPORTANT INFORMATION
In the unlikely event that any of the following occurs, please contact
[us] immediately. . . . Do not proceed with the procedure.
the donor number on the vial does not match your order;
the racial color code identification on the vial cap does not match
your order;
the color of vial cap and color of the cane do not match . . . [All
punctuation from the original.][49]

This text is followed by an exhortation to contact the sperm bank's genetic counselor for guidance if any of the "unlikely events" mentioned above occurs. One can also circumvent the process of sorting through "racial" characteristics by using the services of a company like "The Scandinavian Cryobank," a Seattle-based semen bank that offers exclusively the semen of Scandinavian donors.[50]

While we think of both racial distinctions and the desire to have children who "match" us as natural, they are the legacy of racist politics that order our lives to the present day. Race, again, is a socio-political category, not a "biological" one. Regarding the racism of this normative desire to have children racially like ourselves, law professor Patricia Williams muses on the decision in the "Baby M." surrogacy case. In Baby M., it was decided that the spermatic father (William Stern) had parental rights that overrode those of the "surrogate" mother (Mary Beth Whitehead), based on Judge Sorkow's supposition that it is natural for people to want children "like" themselves.

> What this reasoning raised for me was an issue of what exactly constituted this likeness? (What would have happened, for example, if Mary Beth Whitehead had turned out to have been the "passed" descendent of [a black ancestor]? What if the child she bore had turned out to be recessively and visibly black? Would the sperm of Stern have been so powerful as to make this child "his" with the exclusivity that Judge Sorkow originally assigned?) What constitutes, moreover, the collective understanding of "unlikeness"?[51]

"Bad" Mothers

Indeed, the assumption that we want children who resemble us is tied up in the history of patrilinealism that demands female conjugal fidelity in order to assure the passage of property to her husband's "blood" heirs.[52] It is particularly strong in the United States where, as a "nation of immigrants," identity is understood to rest heavily on one's ancestry. The social control of women and the enforcement of legal marriage necessitated by such an arrangement continue to be pervasive social facts. Lest this all seem long ago and far away, anthropologist Anna Tsing demonstrates that notions of nurturant motherhood, so prevalent to this day, are still defined and sustained by the constant procreation and circulation of the Good Mother's monstrous Other(s).[53]

The valuation of bodies, sexuality, and children is overdetermined by racialized and sexualized ideologies of good and bad mothers. Good mothers are constructed as white, moneyed, married, monogamous or asexual, sober, selfless, and domestic. Conversely, "bad" mothers are stereotyped as the mirror opposites of "good" mothers: black, poor, unmarried, promiscuous, drug-taking, selfish, inadequately domestic, and, yes, lesbian mothers. One might wonder what all the women who fall under the categorical construct of "bad" mother might possibly have in common. Tsing explains,

> Stories of inappropriate mothering are built from diverse symbolic resources. What brings them together is their cultural opposition as "unnatural" alternatives to more appropriate forms of womanhood and ma-

ternity. By setting a "bad example," these women, in all their diversity, direct those who hear their stories toward the singular path of propriety.[54]

The face of the "bad" mother has changed over time, but there have always been groups of women in the United States who were deemed unworthy of motherhood and whose children were removed by the state. Children were removed on many grounds, "including race and condition of bondage, class, religion, and marital status."[55]

> Throughout American history, the particular populations of women whose motherhood status was vulnerable have shifted. But across time, the girls and women whose motherhood claims were ignored or denied shared a profound vulnerability, because they were defined as *possessing* attributes that counted as social demerits—qualities that marked them as non-mothers. Denial of their motherhood status was also fundamentally a result of what these women *lacked:* rights.[56]

In their opposition to "good" mothers and mothering, all other kinds of ("bad") mothering are collapsed in a field of often mutually inter-changeable discourses around sex, race, poverty, femininity, and other normative ideologies.[57]

Stereotypes do not emerge in isolation. They are always pieces of an intricate discursive machinery of stereotypical figures, which only make sense in relation to one another. The iconography and ideology of domestic womanhood and motherhood were consonant with the needs of capitalist chattel-slavery. The idealized mother figure constructed through religious, medical, legal, and popular discourses in eighteenth- and nineteenth-century America was by definition racially white, while black womanhood under slavery was constructed as the white woman's mirror opposite: "impure," wanton, non-domestic, physically strong, anti-family, bestial. These stereotypes are mutually dependent, if unequally destructive. As Donna Haraway writes, "Race and gender are about en-twined, barely analytically separable, highly protean, *relational* categories" (emphasis Haraway's).[58]

Medicine has contributed to such discourses through the medical cate-gorization of "deviant" women as pathological.

> In late Victorian American medicine, degeneration theory was an essen-tial element in linking a wide variety of marginalized women. Social

and medical condemnations of these individuals were strengthened by their links to each other, forming an interwoven network of "degenerate" groups and classifications.[59]

While the "deviant" woman and the "bad" mother are configured in less explicitly medicalized language today, they are still powerful cultural tropes that function to maintain social hierarchies and keep women in line.

In response to such powerful discourses, women create and use complex strategies of resistance to the (symbolic and legislated) dehumanization that they routinely experience. Women, in various ways, make efforts to gain legitimacy and rights in the face of pervasive narratives with predetermined outcomes.

Perhaps intentional lesbian mothers are not recuperable into existing discourses of womanhood and motherhood. The lesbian AI mother is neither virgin nor whore, unwed (read: poor) mother or non-mother.[60] Nor is she a culturally and legally approved mother. Nor is she a putatively heterosexual "single mother," which is, as anthropologist Ellen Lewin observed, a category in transition. The old stigmatized discourse populated by "unwed mothers," "divorcees," and "broken homes" does not quite fit. But neither does the "single mother" escape the modifier "single" that separates her from those in the unmarked, and therefore normative, category of "mother" with all the assumptions of propriety, goodness, and femininity fulfilled that it carries.[61] In this unrecuperable aspect, lesbian marriage and motherhood disrupt foundational cultural myths.

Alternative insemination is a product of its historical and ideological context, even as, in its lesbian forms, it deeply challenges the sex-gender-kinship status quo. Lesbians, along with everyone else, draw from the symbolics of our cultures to make our lives and their meanings. Oppressed people do not generally have the luxury of rejecting outright the culture of those who oppress them. Rather, as Chicana lesbian scholar and activist Gloria Anzaldúa points out in a different context, oppressed people often have to tolerate ambiguity, to take what is forced onto them and adapt it to their own needs.[62] To paraphrase a Marxian formulation, modes of resistance come not from a source external to the culture, but from the contradictions and fissures in the ideology of the culture itself. The culture provides the opportunities (and terms) for its own resistance.

3

Disfertile Discourses
The Inability of Infertility Medicine
to Conceive of Lesbian Mothering

ABSTRACT

In this chapter, I argue that women's, and particularly lesbians', self-inseminating is threatening to male power, speaks of female prerogatives to procreate without men, and is therefore still stigmatized in medical discourse and practice. Further, I demonstrate that medical hegemony over "fertility" powerfully affects the lives of inseminating lesbians.

Biomedicalized AI—Lesbians Negotiate the Fertility Complex

In medical sociologist Laura Mamo's study of "achieving pregnancy in the absence of heterosexuality," Mamo observes and interviews lesbians who wish to inseminate, are in the process of inseminating, or have already inseminated.[1] She finds that they negotiate the medical, social, and ethical terrain of sperm selection with eyes wide open. These women are sensitive to the multiple issues involved and engage in constant self-reflection and discussion. Responding to obstacles they encounter, inseminating lesbians continually revise their initial plans and priorities throughout the process of achieving pregnancy.

For the lesbians in Mamo's study, achieving pregnancy was highly medicalized. "The social status of being a 'lesbian' is translated into a 'biomedical' infertility factor that facilitates movement into biomedicine to seek solutions to an otherwise social problem."[2]

Alternative insemination must be understood vis-à-vis the historic relationship between women (lesbians, mothers) and the male-dominated medical establishment. One reason AI is such an informative site of sociological knowledge is that it participates in all the sexual politics of medicine that permeate our (gendered) relationships with our bodies and with the scientific disciplines.[3]

The medical profession is still a male-dominated elite with a cultural and legal monopoly over medical practice in most countries, including over AI. At the same time, the gender composition of the medical profession is changing profoundly, with many medical school classes equal by sex. It will still take a long time before those with the most institutional power in the medical establishment are not overwhelmingly male. Even with the influx of women medical students and physicians beginning in the 1970s, the norms, standards, beliefs, medical models, and orientation of the professional culture are still male-made and male-defined. Doctors in their offices perform the overwhelming majority of inseminations, and in many countries (and in at least twenty-three states in the United States) it is illegal for AI to be performed by anyone except a licensed physician.[4] In Georgia, the penalty for a non-physician who performs AI is one to five years in prison. In Idaho, a woman who conceives through AI is required by law to inform the physician who attends her birth that she conceived with AI.

The biomedical model underlying the medical establishment emphasizes heroic interventions into the health problems of individuals. Rather than emphasizing public health or other ecosystem approaches (e.g., primary prevention, international health policy, body-mind medicine, community health, occupational safety, environmentalism), the medical establishment is built on the model of radical individualism. In this paradigm, the physician is a kind of secular high priest, whose special knowledge enables him or her to perform heroic interventions into health crises. The continuing medical emphasis on the heroism of the physician diminishes the ecosystem branches of the medical system in favor of a more atomized, commodified, and linear narrative of illness and cure. In the case of infertility, this individualistic bias is brought into sharp relief by the massive medical focus on the "ageless agony" of childlessness, to the neglect of the health needs of those who are already pregnant or postpartum, and of children who are already born. The politics of the biomedical model, also known as the "male medical model," have been widely criticized by many in the overlapping groups of feminists, disability rights activists, sociologists, activists for communities of color, and others.[5]

Medicalization, Demedicalization

Medicalization is a major component of the expansion of medical social control. Medicalization has been defined as "a process by which non-medical problems become defined and treated as medical problems, usually in terms of illnesses or disorders."[6] Although this definition accepts more than I might that things coming under physicians' purview are even problems, the process whereby greater and greater areas of human life come under the authority of medicine is found throughout family life, lesbian and gay as well as straight. Birth has been moved to the hospital even though it is usually low-risk.[7] Sexuality is the site of numerous technological and psychiatric interventions aimed at producing a "healthy" (normative) sexuality.[8] And women's bodies have been pathologized and "treated" as inherently sick or sickening depending on the woman's socioeconomic status.[9] Each of these arenas has seen active struggles for demedicalization and "patient power" by progressive political movements.

The late sociologist and disability rights activist Irving Kenneth Zola found four widespread processes through which medicalization expands and becomes normalized:

> [F]irst, through the expansion of what in life is deemed relevant to the good practice of medicine; secondly, through the retention of absolute control over certain technical procedures; third, through the retention of absolute access to certain "taboo" areas; and finally, through the expansion of what in medicine is deemed relevant to good practice of life.[10]

All four of these processes are present in medical AI.[11] In the case of AI, calls for demedicalization may also be calls for lesbian empowerment.

The dominance of the medical model of AI remained unchallenged until the 1970s, when lesbians using AI began to appropriate formerly taboo AI technologies. The demedicalized lesbian practices of AI bear little resemblance to medical practices, and use radically different language to describe themselves.

The demedicalization of AI began in the late 1960s with the feminist and patients' self-help movements. It emerged from political movements that strove to demystify medicine and seize power from the hands of physicians and the medical system. Emerging from the feminist movement, women's investigations of AI were consonant with practices and discourses around self-empowerment, self-help, and female autonomy. Just as women were fighting political battles for abortion rights, sexual freedom, and other forms of bodily self-determination, many women believed that the choice of when and how to have children should be up to them, independent of the patriarchal norms and standards of the medical profession or the heteropatriarchal family.

It became apparent that the practice of AI was not dependent on medical intervention. Rather, it was readily available to any fertile woman with an eyedropper and a little semen. The self-inseminator's problem is less medical than practical—where can she get the sperm she needs to have the baby she wants? This problem is only medical inasmuch as it is technical—the sperm needs to be kept warm (but not too warm) and used quickly.

The proliferation of successful self-insemination shows that for a healthy woman, physician participation in AI is generally medically unnecessary. Unembellished AI, using untreated semen, is quite straightforward. Members of the Boston Women's Health Book Collective, pioneers of the women's health movement and gynecological self-exam, describe its relative ease:

> [Alternative insemination] is the simplest, least invasive and most widely used of the [procreative technologies]. It doesn't require professional help, and we can do it at home . . . [B]egin by charting your basal temperature and mucus consistency for a few months so that you know when you are likely to ovulate. You must also find a fertile man who is willing to donate sperm. You can do this yourself or, if you want anonymity, through a friend. When you know from past cycles that you are about to ovulate, the sperm donor must masturbate into a clean . . . jar. Within an hour after ejaculation, you suck the semen into a needleless hypodermic syringe (some women use an eye dropper or a turkey baster), gently insert the syringe into your vagina while lying flat on your back with your rear up on a pillow and empty the syringe into

your vagina to deposit the semen as close to your cervix as possible. Then continue lying down comfortably for about ten minutes, so that as little sperm as possible leaks out of your vagina . . . Most women become pregnant after trying [AI] during three to five cycles.[12]

Although they go on to discuss medical screening, anonymity, the costs of going through doctors, and legal questions, the authors' emphasis on the simplicity and speed of the process reminds the reader that this is a woman-controlled process she can trust her body to perform.

Other feminist and/or lesbian publications also emphasize the ease, effectiveness, low cost (potentially no cost if one already owns a thermometer and an eyedropper), and autonomy of AI. Members of the Santa Cruz Women's Health Collective write,

Contrary to what we've been told, the mechanics of alternative fertilization are as easy as 1-2-3. (1) The donor ejaculates into a clean small jar or into a condom. (2) The semen is delivered to the woman. (3) Lying down, she transfers the semen to her vagina, using an eyedropper, a turkey baster, diaphragm, etc., or inserts the inverted condom.[13]

The authors acknowledge, "[t]hings other than the actual mechanics aren't quite so simple. Finding a donor, estimating the time of ovulation, and dealing with emotional factors."[14] Yet, significantly, none of these three "things" falls within the medical domain. Alternative insemination is again a process controlled by the woman.

The existence of such demedicalized (and differently medicalized) practices challenges the medical monopoly over AI, and reduces the power of physicians and the medical profession to exert social control by dictating the terms of who shall and shall not become pregnant. Because of the demonstrated social conservatism and prejudices of the medical profession in this area, this demedicalization further democratizes access to AI.[15] The presence of economic and professional competitors on the scene pulls the medical establishment toward liberalization of its own selection processes. If women can simply get semen from a friend, or a friendly sperm bank, then infertility specialists and family physicians are motivated by their own financial self-interests to accept a more diverse clientele. In fact, more and more infertility doctors have accepted lesbian and single women AI "patients" since the 1980s. (Other factors have influenced this shift in physician attitudes as well.) While the counter-current created by self-insemination has not changed the values or practices of most physicians, it offers a positive and self-perpetuating force of resistance as the infrastructure for lesbian insemination expands.

Physicians may or may not provide ancillary benefits to the inseminee, such as medical screening of sperm donors, legal protections from sperm donor challenges to lesbian family integrity, privacy, medical options if the woman's fertility is a problem, and, perhaps, psychological reassurance. One recent U.S. study found that lesbian inseminees and their partners cited a concern for medical safety and fear of a known donor intruding into their families, as well as the obvious desire to have a child, as the top reasons for wanting to inseminate in a medical setting. As for procuring the sperm and performing the insemination, the woman herself, a friend, or a lover could just as easily replace the physician.[16]

For lesbians, AI is not a treatment for a medical condition. Rather, it is a procreative option for women who wish to become mothers. This paradigmatic difference is borne out in the feminist literature on self-insemination, which places AI in the context of the range of issues facing lesbians and/or single women who want to become mothers.[17]

While the emergence of a lucrative and high-tech semen-banking industry may make self-insemination seem passé, many lesbians still practice it.[18] At-home self-insemination is the non-medical standard against which to compare its practice in the medical establishment. Yet for most of its relatively short history, AI has been securely under the purview and power of physicians.[19]

If we place two designations, "medical" and "non-medical," on the ends of a continuum, some inseminations will take place on either pole, and others will partake of at least some of each opposite.[20] In the middle of the spectrum, we might find feminist health centers where nurse practitioners do medical screening of donors and recipients but orient their services toward lesbian clients. While the medical and non-medical designations are necessarily reductive, they allow discussion of important differences in how insemination is performed and experienced, as well as in the meanings that are made from the process.

The non-medical practice of AI is rather simple, physiologically if not socio-legally. Non-medical AI encompasses the laywomen who for themselves and each other obtain the sperm to self-inseminate. It also includes literature, writings, web sites, and self-help networks that help women self-inseminate outside the medical setting. On the other hand, even the ostensibly "low tech" practices of AI often require a sophisticated understanding of female reproductive physiology and the ability to track and predict fertile windows of opportunity for insemination.

One example is the use of ovulation-prediction kits (OPK). While these kits are sold at the local drugstore and promise to be "easy" and "accurate," the truth is more complicated. In a chapter called "Hatching and Catching the Egg," Mohler and Frazer describe some of the many factors that can go wrong when using ovulation-predictor kits.[21] Inaccurate results might be caused by menopause or fertility medications, or by excessive or inadequate amount or density of urine on the test. Reading the results can be tricky since colors can change over the course of the several minutes the test is supposed to be readable, leaving some guesswork to the woman. Moreover, the woman is supposed to take the test during her "peak period," which she must determine, and then take the test at the same time each afternoon over the course of several days. The tests are also an extra expense. The final point on Mohler and Frazer's list of concerns emerges as a culmination of all of these: "Difficulties in interpreting the test results can be 'extremely stressful.'" Mohler and Frazer conclude with the caveat that the OPK "can provide valuable information *when used in combination with the other prediction/ovulation tracking methods.*" Although they have gotten easier to use since these words were written, the OPK is not the "simple," "easy," or necessarily "accurate" technology its advertisers would have us believe.[22]

The medical practice of AI includes the infertility specialists and other physicians who offer AI services through their medical practices, and also the professional literature, norms, sperm banks, clinics, and organizations (e.g., the American College of Obstetricians and Gynecologists) that make up the medical establishment providing AI-related services. It also includes the literature by and about infertile couples and their struggles to have babies, including with AI. Often these are heart-rending accounts of the agonizing pain suffered by infertile couples.[23] While these texts are personal, intimate, and non-scientific, I put them in the medical camp because they stem from, and respond to, a medical condition (infertility).[24] While fairly diverse, this literature generally does not challenge the hegemony of the medical system as the appropriate provider of AI. Nor does it challenge assumptions about universal heterosexuality and ideologies of fertility (e.g., any woman seeking AI does so as a response to male infertility) that underlie the medical discourses.

AI and Infertility

The medical discourse about AI places it securely in the company of other medical treatments of infertility. Alternative insemination is seen to be on the non-intrusive end of a continuum of medical techniques that might benefit "the infertile couple" as it has been constructed within discourses of patriarchal biofamilism. Alternative insemination, fertility drugs, intrauterine insemination (IUI), gamete intrafallopian transfer (GIFT), zygote intrafallopian transfer (ZIFT), in vitro fertilization (IVF), intracytoplasmic sperm injection (ICSI), and "surrogate motherhood" are some practices in the domain of the fertility specialist. Among this assemblage, AI is understood as a treatment for male infertility. Male infertility is described as follows by the American Society for Reproductive Medicine (ASRM):

> A variety of sperm problems can account for male infertility. Sperm can be completely absent in the ejaculate (azoospermia) or present in low concentrations (oligospermia). They may have poor motility (asthenospermia) or an increased percentage of abnormal shapes and forms (teratospermia). There may also be abnormalities in the series of steps required for fertilization, such as sperm binding to and penetrating the egg. Deficiencies in any of these aspects of sperm function will generally lead to lack of fertilization.[25]

While the numbers are contested, the general consensus suggests that approximately 8.5 percent (or one in twelve) of U.S. married couples in their "childbearing years" are infertile, with infertility defined as "the inability to conceive after a year or more of sexual relations [sic] without contraception."[26] Infertility is not equally distributed across countries, or even within countries, but rather correlates strongly with poverty.[27]

Fertility specialists are motivated, financially and professionally, to use higher-intervention methods, and a woman who goes to a fertility specialist for AI is more likely to have her situation medicalized than one who inseminates at home or in the intermediary space of a feminist or lesbian health center. Fertility doctors are likely to see the woman who wants to get pregnant as having a medical problem. Most of their experience, practice, and gaze is heteronormative and concerned with the infertility problems of heterosexual couples.

This orientation may be a blessing for a woman who has fertility problems and desires medical intervention. But for lesbians without fertility problems, it is more often a curse. Fertility treatments such as intrauterine insemination (IUI), sperm-washing, fertility drugs, and IVF all have helped women to get pregnant who would be unable to do so with AI alone.[28] On the other hand, for healthy women with no fertility problems, fertility technology may be unnecessarily interventionist. A lesbian seeing fertility doctors may be subjected to intrusive and medically unnecessary "screenings" or mandatory psychiatric testing and counseling, paid for by the client. Sperm-washing and intrusive insemination techniques such as IUI are other treatments that gate-keeping doctors may impose. In an anomalous case, I spoke with a woman whose physician pressured her to undergo ICSI even though she was perfectly fertile.[29] The general orientation of fertility doctors to heroic interventions in the "desperately" infertile make the likelihood of inappropriate treatments high. Dealing with such interventions, whether by undergoing or resisting them, often takes a toll on a lesbian's emotional and/or physical well-being.

Those doctors most likely to perform AI, whether they are family doctors or andrologists, gynecologists or endocrinologists, have a stake in the social construction of infertility. Infertility can, of course, be caused by any number of factors, with male- and female-factor infertility occurring more or less equally. In about 20 percent of cases, physicians are unable to discover any cause(s) of the infertility.[30] In those heterosexual couples where the male is infertile, the woman's reproductive system is usually perfectly healthy, and vice versa. In other words, a married man's fertility problem is not automatically transmitted to his wife.

Yet "the infertile couple" is the subject of extensive research, experimentation, and "treatment." This inability to distinguish between a woman's body and that of her husband is further displayed by two descriptors in the medical AI lexicon, which are used as exhaustive and mutually exclusive categories: "homologous AI" and "heterologous AI." "Homologous AI" refers to AIH (alternative insemination by husband) while "heterologous AI" refers to AID (alternative insemination by donor).

Yet, plainly, any sperm a woman takes into her body is by definition "different" from and external to her body before insemination. The idea that marriage renders a husband's sperm "homologous" to his wife displays the patriarchal ideology of the medical establishment (with the complete cooperation of the law) that diminishes the subjectivity of women as soon as marriage or procreation is raised. This suppression of female subjectivity is perhaps most visible in the rituals of patriarchal marriage in which the bride loses her name, her property becomes her husband's, and even her selfhood may (legally and culturally) be subsumed into the identity of her husband.[31] The discursive erasure of lesbian existence is also achieved by the medical language of "homologous" and "heterologous" AI, since the only options these terms permit require that a woman seeking insemination be married and that the semen come from either her husband or an extramarital "other."

Some physicians who refuse to inseminate lesbians justify this on the same basis that insurance carriers justify the decision only to cover married women: that they treat infertility, and when a woman in a married couple seeks AI, it is because of infertility "in the couple" (e.g., the husband is infertile) or because of a medical problem "in the couple" that requires "treatment" (e.g., a child born to that couple would have a high risk of Hodgkin's disease).[32] This line of reasoning could easily be extended to lesbians who wish to become pregnant, whose (female) partners are unable to impregnate them, thus constituting another type of "infertile couple"—the socially infertile rather than the medically infertile.[33] That lesbian couples are not considered "infertile couples" can be seen as yet another instance of medical heterosexism.

The Catholic Church and other conservative religious denominations share this apparent lack of sympathy toward the inability of same-sex couples to procreate through their normal sexual activities. Conservative gay pundit Andrew Sullivan explains, "the Catholic Church affirms that the sexual act [sic] must be both 'procreative,' i.e., open to baby making, and 'unitive,' i.e., loving." That same-sex couples are physiologically barred from the former, he argues, should not also bar them from the latter, or from the sacrament of marriage. He holds up infertile heterosexual couples as analogous to same-sex couples in this respect (their sexuality may be loving, but not procreative) and remarks on the sympathy and compassion shown to infertile heterosexual couples, who are allowed by the church to marry and have sex. He then asks why the same opportunity is denied to homosexuals, who may equally "long to have unitive and procreative sex; and to have children. They are just tragically unable, as the Church sees it, to experience the joy of a procreative married life."[34]

"The truth is," Sullivan laments, "as the current doctrine now stands, the infertile are defined by love and compassion, while homosexuals are defined by loneliness and sin. The Church has no good case why this should be so."[35] Neither, I would add, do the medical or insurance establishments. Sadly, however, no "good case" need be made by the Catholic hierarchy, nor, only slightly more surprisingly, must it be made in the halls of Congress, or in the supposedly less partisan setting of a doctor's office.[36] Yet while the medical profession has rarely hesitated to pathologize lesbians as both physiologically and psychologically ill, in/fertility seems to be a rare case when lesbians are not deemed to have a medical problem.[37] Lesbian fertility issues remain invisible in this discourse, since the infertile are assumed to be heterosexual.

Profitable Infertility

Medical AI is not cheap. Health insurance providers are only mandated to cover infertility services in ten U.S. states, and mandated to offer them in three.[38] While these laws vary from state to state, all of them require infertility as a prerequisite for access. When regulating insurance coverage for access to treatment for infertility, relatively inexpensive AI is not a main focus of the laws; in vitro fertilization (IVF) is. Three of the states that mandate infertility coverage (Arkansas, Hawaii, and Maryland) mandate only coverage for IVF, and one (Texas) mandates offering only IVF coverage. In each of these states, and in the more comprehensive policy of Illinois, access to IVF in particular has many stipulations, including that the patient's eggs be fertilized by her husband's sperm.[39] Needless to

say, no Arkansan insurance company will be required by the state to provide reproductive services to lesbians, regardless of how well insured they
are. Lesbians will pay out-of-pocket for all other infertility services as
well. Only Illinois, Massachusetts, and New Jersey specifically mandate
coverage for AI for the infertile, though access to it would seem also to
fall under the general provisions of Montana, Rhode Island, and West
Virginia and to be offered in California and Connecticut.

Defining infertility then becomes the crux of the matter. In most cases,
defining infertility follows a timetable of unprotected (implicitly heterosexual) sex. California defines it with two possibilities: a demonstrated
medical condition or inability to conceive or carry a pregnancy after a year
of unprotected sexual activity without contraception. Connecticut and
Illinois define it as being either unable to get pregnant or unable to carry
a pregnancy to term over the course of a year. In New Jersey, infertility's
definition varies by age of the patient: It is the inability to get pregnant
after two years for a woman under 35 and one year for a woman over 35.
In a gender neutral twist, Massachusetts defines it as being unable to
conceive or produce conception during a one-year period. Only Rhode
Island defines infertility exclusively as the condition of a married individual unable to conceive or produce conception during a period of a
year. Montana and West Virginia do not define infertility or the scope of
services offered.

The promotion of infertility as a disease expands the market for medical infertility services. This expansion is part of the larger problem of
commodified health and health care in the United States. As medical sociologists Peter Conrad and Rochelle Kern explain:

> The medical industries . . . have turned certain goods and services into
> products or commodities that can be marketed to meet "health needs"
> created by the industry itself . . . A wide range of products have been
> marketed to meet commodified health needs, such as products designed
> to alleviate feminine hygiene "problems" and instant milk formulas to
> meet the "problem" of feeding infants.[40]

High infertility rates lead to increased funding for research into treatments. These treatments in turn are offered to more and more women,
thus reinforcing the expectation that women will subject themselves to

infertility "treatments," which expands the market, and so on in an extremely lucrative upward spiral. Two percent of U.S. women of "childbearing age" have made a medical visit for infertility in the past year, and 8 percent have made such a visit in their lifetimes.[41] That translates into nearly five million "heterosexual" U.S. couples in which the female partner is 15 to 44 years of age reporting difficulty or delay in achieving a live birth, and 1.3 million receiving medical advice or treatment for infertility yearly.[42] These are massive numbers, especially when one thinks of the painful, expensive, experimental, and risky treatments involved.

The infertility establishment seems as sinister as any other large profit-motivated industry when one realizes that both infertility rates and individual infertility diagnoses are determined by how infertility is defined. As Harvard biologist Ruth Hubbard points out, the one-year standard for infertility is arbitrarily (read: profitably) short. In other countries, infertility is figured differently. In France, for example, a heterosexual couple must "try" for two years before infertility is diagnosed. Since many babies are conceived in the second year, France has lower infertility rates than the United States.[43]

The infertility industry has been critiqued at length for its apparent disregard for women's well-being, abuse of animals in "experimentation" and factory farming, dishonest sales tactics, inflated success rates, high cost, and general misrepresentation of what it can offer. Fertility societies such as the ASRM acknowledge these problems in their updated guidelines for the practice of fertility medicine, in which they recommend against excesses such as denying patients informed consent and misrepresenting success rates.[44] As they delicately phrase it:

> With the proliferation of ART programs and the recent controversy concerning the numerous United States IVF programs reported to have little or no success, it was believed appropriate to issue an updated set of minimum standards for ART programs.[45]

The ASRM uses the standard medical definition of infertility: "Infertility is a disease that exists when a couple has tried to conceive for 12 months during which time they have had intercourse [sic] without the use of contraception."[46] This definition has several problems. Infertility may or may not be caused by a disease. Certainly the woman who receives (insurance reimbursed) AI based on her husband's infertility does not have a disease. Nor do lesbians, who may want to inseminate, have a disease. The American Psychiatric Association (APA) declassified homosexuality as a mental illness in 1973 and the World Health Organization (WHO) deleted homosexuality from its International Classification of Diseases twenty years later, in January of 1993.[47] Rather, it is the discourse of the medical establishment, mired in heteropatriarchal assumptions, that apparently cannot see anything but disease when it looks at an "infertile couple" or unhusbanded (including lesbian) woman.

Framing infertility in this manner discursively undermines healthy women viewing AI as a procreative option. The fact that many perfectly fertile lesbians and other unmarried women seek out AI is made invisible by the "disease" model of insemination. The medical establishment defines its market as exclusively "infertile (heterosexual) couples," even though the existence of inseminating lesbians is well known, or certainly should be, by those involved with AI. Yet the infertility establishment, whose self-interest is not hard to ascertain, pities, medicalizes, and marginalizes all non-procreatively coupled women, and offers technological salvation in the form of instrumental and contractual procreation. In *From the Beginning: A History of the American Fertility Society 1944–1994,* the volume commemorating the fiftieth anniversary of its founding, the ASRM declares its "dedication . . . to resolving the ageless agony of childlessness and other reproductive illnesses."[48]

At the risk of belaboring the obvious: Since when has childlessness been an illness?[49] What about the ageless agony of women's and (to a large extent) men's lives being consumed by unplanned pregnancies and children? While the ASRM also acclaims its role in the creation of oral contraception ("The Pill"), this historic accomplishment receives short shrift when compared to the society's pride in its role in developing ART.[50]

While the emotional pain of many infertile people is well documented, it is not universal. A variety of factors make it impossible to determine the prevalence of a distraught response to learning of, and living with, one's infertility. These factors include the following.

- Those who would not mind being infertile probably practice some form of birth control, and so may never learn of their infertility.

- Those who are very distraught about their infertility are the most vocal (though the converse, that those who are the most vocal are the most upset, is not necessarily true).
- People who are not especially upset are less likely to publicize their infertility.
- Subjective reactions to infertility are profoundly shaped by the cultural context of the physical and psychological difficulty of infertility treatment and the expense and difficulty of adoption.

Still, we know that hundreds of thousands of people each year make medical infertility visits, that millions of dollars are spent each year on infertility treatments, and that psychological and social support resources for the emotional pain of involuntary childlessness are in high demand.[51]

The promotion of the trope, and treatment, of the "tragic barren woman" (now in her modern, medicalized guise as the "infertility patient"), however, is more than a canny economic move on behalf of physicians. As anthropologist Susan Martha Kahn points out, the idea that barrenness is the ultimate form of female suffering is as ancient as the lament of biblical matriarch Rachel: "Give me sons or else I am dead."[52] This discourse perpetuates the ancient, sexist assumption that in a heterosexual couple, infertility is the woman's "fault." It is also part of the ideology that pressures women into heterosexuality, marriage, and motherhood, while marginalizing lesbians as beyond the pale of motherhood. That these same fertility "experts" have historically refused to help inseminate lesbians who request it further exposes the cynicism of their stance.[53]

This double standard, by which the infertility industry reifies and reinforces the tragic infertility of heterosexual women, also trivializes and pathologizes the desire of non-heterosexual women to have children. The dominance of the heteropatriarchal family model marks a sharp dichotomy in the treatment of women by the infertility establishment. If the experience of infertility is a tragedy, as it certainly is for many, then the infertility of lesbians is no less tragic. The challenges lesbians face getting pregnant may be different from those of heterosexual women, or they may be the same. But while doctors pathologize both lesbians and heterosexual women, those heterosexual women who have health insurance are almost endlessly "helped" to have babies, whereas lesbians' fertility needs typically have been consigned to the margins of the infertility specialist's screen. The fact that a lesbian desires to have a child at all is still often seen as pathology. This view is counteracted, however, by the fact that in today's world of puny reimbursements for straight women's infertility services, lesbians pay cash.

Lesbian Invisibility

The idea of erasure is important to feminist and postcolonial literary theory and cultural studies. Erasure is not exactly oppression or suppression, but rather being eliminated from the field of language, not being heard. Certain narratives are told over and over, making some realities visible while erasing others. This process is at the heart of political struggles over defining the canon and who gets to be part of the official story and who does not. Invisibility, erasure, and closeting all connect to the denial of the history of lesbian mothers. The silence about lesbian AI and lesbian mothering echoes through the discourses that constitute our official knowledge of procreation, sexual activity, household composition, and family makeup in this country.

For instance, the OTA used to conduct studies and authorize reports on an array of complex technological issues that the Congress deemed relevant. These reports were used by members of Congress and others as authoritative scientific documents that adhered to the most effective, accurate, and current methodologies to make objective assessments of (usually medical, social, or technological) issues. This was the last U.S. federal agency that studied or reported on alternative insemination.

The OTA's last publication relevant to lesbian AI is the *Report of the National Survey of Family Growth* (NSFG). The NSFG is "a multipurpose survey based on personal interviews with a national sample of women 15–44 years of age in the civilian noninstitutionalized population of the United States. Its main function is to collect data on factors affecting pregnancy and women's health in the United States."[54] Previous NSFG surveys were conducted in 1973, 1976, 1982, 1988, and 1990.[55] This report, conducted in 1995 under the auspices of the National Institutes of Health (NIH), contains data on a wide range of topics related to women's health and procreating. Topics include the number of children women have had and the number they expect in the future, intended and unintended births, "sexual intercourse," marriage and cohabitation, infertility, impaired fecundity and sterilization operations, breastfeeding, maternity leave and child care, adoption, stepchildren and foster children, health insurance coverage, family planning, and other medical services.[56]

This is exactly the type of social science research that could tell us a lot about lesbians and their families, including the use of AI in family building. Lesbians are involved in every one of the above categories. Yet if one read this document without knowing better, one might surmise that no lesbian, bisexual, or gay man lived in this country. Alternative insemination, which is difficult to discuss without including lesbians, is subsumed under the category of "infertility." The 125-page report of this massive longitudinal study has not one word about lesbians, homosexuality, gay women, women cohabiting, or anything else that might indicate that the existence of lesbians is more prevalent than the existence of, say, unicorns. Even while the study claims to document the diversity of kinship, sexual, and procreative arrangements in the United States, it reaffirms heteronormativity as the single possibility that exists, or is even imaginable. Lesbian invisibility is a factor that works against the protection of lesbian rights throughout the world.[57] As the International Lesbian and Gay Human Rights Commission reports,

> Not only do most violations of lesbians' human rights (like violations of women's rights more generally) take place within the "private" sphere, but also the silence that surrounds lesbianism adds an additional layer of difficulty in documenting such violations. For example, the barriers that keep women from reporting domestic violence or rape—shame, fear, lack of appropriate services—are well known. Those barriers are even higher when reporting an incident requires that a woman admit to the police or other authorities that she is a lesbian.[58]

Whether or not explicit prohibitions against lesbianism exist in the law, women put themselves at great risk—jeopardizing family relationship, friendships, physical safety, employment, and housing—if they publicly acknowledge that they are lesbians. Most lesbians must also contend with the self-doubt and shame that widespread prejudice engenders. The rules may be unwritten—or even unspoken—but they are real, and the official silence surrounding lesbianism only makes it harder to document, respond to, or resist the abuses that lesbians experience.[59]

While lesbians are increasingly visible in many countries, as gay, lesbian, and bisexual people emerge into a cultural milieu undeniably changed by feminist and queer movements, the closet remains powerful, and is bound up in foundational metaphysical binaries that shape our consciousness and culture.[60] The power of the closet, and the erasures it enacts, enables those involved in contractual and technological procreation to deny the centrality of lesbians to their enterprise.

Medicalization and invisibility work together to disempower lesbians under the sign of taboo. This effect is documented vividly by anthropologist Kath Weston, who notes that older books about homosexuality in the Stanford University library still carry the "locked stack" imprint.[61] Homosexuality itself was both pathologized and made invisible through the social control of knowledge in the organization of the library.

Historian Jennifer Terry documents the medicalization of lesbian existence through the search for signs on and in the (constructed-as-deviant) lesbian body. The species difference attributed to female and male homosexuals was sought and documented in meticulously measured deviations in the dimensions of lesbian nipples, lesbian clitorises, and lesbian psyches.[62] The female "homosexual" has always been defined as medically pathological, unlike the countless women who were erotically involved with other women before the invention ("discovery") of hetero- and homo-sexualities in the nineteenth century. Again, the pathologization of the lesbian as grotesque, and her invisibility, coincide as taboo.[63]

A central aspect of medical social control is its domain over "taboo" areas of life: sexuality, but also women's bodies and processes of procreation.[64] Feminist philosopher Mary Daly describes the prohibition against "women touching women" (lesbian existence) as the "Terrible Taboo":

> Terrible Taboo: the universal, unnatural patriarchal taboo against women Intimately/Ultimately Touching each Other; prohibition stemming from male terror of women who exercise Elemental Touching Powers.[65]

When psychiatry took the helm from pre-Freudian medicine (and as eugenics fell out of favor following World War II), lesbians and other sexual "deviants," as well as all other women, were pathologized by psychiatry rather than by eugenics per se.[66] Pathologization made lesbians rare, exotic, species-different, Other, and at the same time Taboo. Lesbians were inscribed in a "monster story" in which they stood, even if just below consciousness, as a terrifying cautionary tale to women. Lesbians were cast as anti-woman, anti-mother, anti-feminine, anti-family, unnatural, and Godless. Small wonder that doctors, as generators of these discourses, and as recipients of cultural tropes, have resisted lesbian requests for insemination.[67]

It is unacceptable for general practitioners, gynecologists, and fertility specialists to claim to be unaware of the prevalence of lesbian insemination today. Such "ignorance" is politically invested and based on heterosexual privilege.[68] Yet the denial continues and takes numerous shapes.

One rarely sees the word "lesbian" in the medical literature about AI. Yet the existence of lesbian AI intrudes into even the heteronormative world of seemingly lesbian-less medical texts. One must actively search for these references, reading between the lines, much like one must read for lesbian existence in other realms of heterosexist culture such as cinema, TV, music, or history. One example of the almost-visible lesbian can be found in the official magazine of the U.S. Food and Drug Administration, FDA Consumer, in a reference to an insemination practice. Under the sign of infertility, lesbian AI can be sighted if you squint.

> Sometimes it may be necessary or preferable to get pregnant without intercourse [sic]. A woman may choose to get pregnant with the sperm of someone who is not her partner. [Emphasis added.][69]

Lest we get too excited over this possible allusion to lesbian existence, the sentences that immediately follow reassert that the only possible framework for insemination is heterosexual:

> In some cases, a woman may not be able to become pregnant with her partner because his sexual problems make it impossible for him to ejaculate normally during sex, or because the sperm have to bypass the vagina if the vaginal mucus cannot support them, or for other reasons. In these cases, through artificial insemination, the semen is placed into the woman's uterus or vaginal canal. . . .[70]

How different this document would be if the FDA authorized inclusion of a few sentences that reflected the fact of lesbian insemination and lesbian existence:

> Sometimes a woman may not be able to get pregnant with her partner because her partner is also a woman. In these cases alternative insemination is indicated as a first-line therapy.

By retrieving lesbian insemination from the realm of the unspeakable, the FDA could help destigmatize lesbian AI, lesbian families, and lesbians in general. The day that such sentences become included routinely in government documents discussing AI, fertility, family formations, and other related areas will be a happy one indeed.

I could barely believe my eyes when I read the ASRM's current guidelines for AI (which they call therapeutic donor insemination, or TDI), and discovered that lesbians have almost been acknowledged as the major recipients they are.

Indications for TDI
A. The male partner has azoospermia, severe oligospermia, or has other significant sperm or seminal fluid abnormalities.
B. The male partner has a known hereditary or genetic disorder (e.g., Huntington's disease, hemophilia, chromosomal anomalies) that confers a very high risk to biologic offspring.
C. The male partner has noncorrectable ejaculatory dysfunction secondary to trauma, surgery, medication, psychological abnormalities, etc.
D. The female partner is Rh-negative and severely Rh-isoimmunized, and the male partner is Rh-positive.
E. In assisted reproductive technologies (in vitro fertilization, gamete intrafallopian transfer, zygote intrafallopian transfer) where a significant male factor has been demonstrated (i.e., previous failure to fertilize, significant oligoasthenospermia, male immunologic infertility) and ICSI is not elected.
F. *In females without male partners.* [Emphasis added.][71]

A few lines later, the document discusses counseling with the couple receiving AI, or with the woman "if she is single"! This is a huge step forward from previous versions of the document. Given the direction the guidelines are moving in, lesbians may actually be acknowledged as recipients of AI in future versions.

Lesbian invisibility, however widespread, does not reflect lesbian non-existence. Lesbians exist, fall in love, form enduring relationships, and become mothers, all in large numbers. Lesbians, like other women, have many different kinds of involvements with the medical establishment and the infertility industry. In the realm of technological and contractual procreation, lesbians are most visible in their use of alternative insemination. Despite the massive erasure of lesbian existence from public and private discourse, the lesbian baby boom and high-profile media events involving AI and lesbian motherhood (e.g., lesbian rock star Melissa Etheridge's partner giving birth to a baby conceived with rock star David Crosby's sperm) have pointed an occasional spotlight on lesbian AI. Even less visible than lesbian insemination, however, is the centrality of lesbians to the entire enterprise of contractual and technological procreation. Lesbian participation is welcomed, even needed (in part due to the "shortage" of human ova), yet the "L-word" is banished from that shrine to medicalized heteropatriarchy, the infertility clinic.

Anne Pollock highlights this contradiction of lesbian centrality and erasure in "The Queers at the Center of High-Tech Reproduction: A Lesbian Body Sells Her Eggs."[72] In this essay, Pollock recounts and theorizes her own experiences selling her ova to a "reproductive clinic." Her narrative is permeated with lesbians. The author, herself a visible lesbian, encounters lesbians at many steps in her process, including, dramatically, the technician who performs her pelvic ultrasound. In order to collect the $2,000 for her participation, however, the young author must go through a bio-psychosocial screening process. In it, she creates "a eugenically perfect history": heterosexual (though barely sexually active and never without condoms), no IV drug use, no psychiatric history (achievement of this status, she notes, is extremely rare for lesbians growing up in the United States), and "feminine" personality traits, such as a fear of spiders. Quite a (gender) performance, yet a simple deception compared to the psychosocial gymnastics typically required by the closet. While the protocols for egg sale called for lesbians, mental health system survivors, and other "eugenically imperfect" women to be screened out, none of the people Pollock encountered challenged her about her clearly marked queerness. Instead, she found the staff of the reproductive clinic "wavering . . . between tacit heteronormative assumptions and a more conscious refusal to identify the lesbian body before them."[73]

If not for her self-reflective essay, the evidence of lesbian existence in this particular edifice to heteropatriarchy would have vanished (as the traces of lesbian lives have been made to vanish throughout patriarchal history). Only because of the vast labors of lesbian and gay activists a generation before her, and the continuing anti-homophobic work of lesbian, gay, and queer activists and their allies, was the infrastructure in place for Pollock to find an audience for her work and, eventually, a publisher. Sadly, neither she nor any lesbian humanist will likely be paid for her scholarly work on a scale even approaching what she was paid for her eggs.[74]

Medical Anti-Lesbianism

The medical profession has a long and shameful history of persecuting lesbians.[75] The categorization of the homosexual as a biologically deformed species, the psychiatric abuse of lesbians and gay men who were labeled psychologically ill, surgery and shock treatment for lesbians, and the refusal of physicians to inseminate lesbians, are but a few examples of medical social control of lesbians and gay men.[76] Even when physicians and researchers admit they have no empirical basis for denying lesbians AI services, they have typically maintained their right to do so.

A 1984 article in a leading infertility journal, entitled "The Single Woman and Artificial Insemination by Donor," focused on ethical considerations of inseminating "single women," a category under which they included lesbians.[77] The authors report the prevalence of objections to such inseminations, including that "a lesbian mother may influence the child to become homosexual." Implicit in this "objection" is the (eugenic) judgment that a gay child is worse than no child at all. That the birth of a baby who would grow up to be "homosexual" should be feared and prevented, rather than welcomed with celebration, is never explained. The heterosexism implicit in this stance is assumed to be so normative as to require no comment.

The authors later grudgingly acknowledge that they can find no data to support their anti-lesbian prejudices, noting, "A review of the relevant social science research indicates . . . that these and other objections are not supported by the available data."[78] Despite this nod in the direction of reality, the authors conclude, "AID for single women is permissible in *selected* cases" (emphasis added). Lest this statement be mistaken for tolerance of "single" motherhood, the authors hasten to reassure the reader—understood to be another physician—that "the physician has a right to refuse to carry out such requests."[79] While it is clear that much has changed since the 1980s, I am unaware of any studies documenting these changes.

Any physician can arrange to facilitate or perform AI without giving it much thought, either with sperm from a sperm bank or through an informal arrangement. According to Jane Mattes, founder and director of the nationwide organization Single Mothers by Choice (SMC), "Members of SMC across the country have found that in general the medical profession is fairly positive about mature, responsible single women trying to get pregnant by insemination. In some cases, and particularly in more conservative areas of the country, you may find doctors whose personal or religious beliefs make them unwilling to inseminate single women, but in our experience this is not typical of the medical profession as a group."[80] The reader will notice that Mattes is describing physician responses to a particularly privileged group of women—those who appear to physicians to be "mature, responsible"—a group that is likely to include many closeted lesbians, although it probably does not include many "obvious" lesbians.

The fact that AI is unregulated leaves much room for individual discretion and bias in physicians' practices regarding lesbian AI, as well as for idiosyncratic practices and rationales. This large amount of physician discretion, interestingly, parallels the excess of judicial discretion when cases involving lesbian AI are brought to court.

The issue of haphazard regulation of AI is not unique to the United States, but is evident across the globe as well. Political scientist Robert H. Blank studied the regulation of AI in thirty-three countries, and found that

> DI [donor insemination] policy in most countries is the product of a
> patchwork and often haphazard combination of programme and profes-

sional guidelines, committee reports, court rulings and in some cases statutory regulations . . . This divergent and potentially conflicting combination of private and public actions results in ambiguous policy.[81]

Regulation, however, should not be seen as a panacea for lesbians wishing to inseminate. Rather, the content of the regulations, and their implementation, are at least as important to lesbians as whether regulations exist at all.[82] In fact, the lack of coherent regulations, and the frequent lack of enforcement of those that do exist, creates important spaces in which lesbians can inseminate. Given the heterosexist and patriarchal norms of medicine, law, and culture, I doubt regulation of AI (or standardization of existing regulations) would work to the benefit of most lesbians.

Protocols against inseminating single or lesbian women are endorsed by the professional organizations that regulate infertility doctors. For a number of reasons, it is difficult to measure physician compliance with the protocols against inseminating unmarried women. Even physicians who regularly inseminate lesbians and single women may be reluctant to admit it, since some have suffered professional castigation.[83] Still, even if not universally adhered to, such protocols and laws reflect and reinforce social norms and have significant cultural power.

The anti-lesbian position of fertility societies is international. The International Federation of Fertility Societies (IFFS) is the leading international body of fertility specialists. In its own words, it wants to

contribute to the standardization of terminology and evaluation of diagnostic and therapeutic procedures in the field of reproduction. Assisted Reproduction Technology (ART) has raised new questions that have been addressed with wide differences depending on culture, religion, or health policy. Many countries have issued laws or regulations and many others are about to do so. In issuing this "Consensus" on a number of ethical issues about ART, IFFS wants to officialise the world of the professionals themselves.

"The International Consensus on Assisted Procreation," produced by the IFFS, extols what it calls "AIP" or "artificial insemination with partner's sperm."

Ethical evaluation: If there is a medical indication for its practice and the individual evaluation of the case shows a greater expectation of pregnancy with insemination than with programmed coitus, we can consider the technique as ethically acceptable.[84]

Regarding AID it is only slightly less effusive:

> We believe that insemination with donor sperm is ethically acceptable if: There is a medical indication and psychological evaluation for its practice; The normal conditions of anonymity and screening of the donor are met; Frozen sperm samples used have passed the appropriate quarantining for the normal infectious disease such as HIV, hepatitis B and C, and syphilis.[85]

When it comes to the insemination of lesbians, the IFFS at least has the stomach to mention it directly:

> The application of artificial insemination with a donor's semen to women without a partner or lesbian couples constitutes a limit indication which should be analyzed with care.[86]

Note that despite the slim potential of lesbian AI indicated by the above, most lesbians would be unlikely to fulfill the minimal qualifications for "AID" as enumerated in the previous paragraph. First, only by an expanded and atypical definition might a lesbian be considered to have insemination "medically indicated" since she is not considered to be part of the gold standard of an "infertile couple."[87] Second, depending on the evaluation instrument, a lesbian might fail the "psychological evaluation" process simply by virtue of being a lesbian. While homosexuality qua homosexuality is no longer considered a mental illness in the United States, known lesbians are still often considered mentally or emotionally unstable by default.

In a text discussing all aspects of AI, an eminent and widely published physician, Dr. Wilfred Finegold, expressed his opinions about the insemination of "single" women. The reader ought to bear in mind that Dr. Finegold is referring to unmarried (presumably) heterosexual women. He does not mention lesbians even once in his 1976 book (an omission that would be nearly impossible today).

> Since no bona fide unmarried patient has ever approached us for donor insemination, we have found this consternation regarding the association

of AI and spinsterhood rather confusing. It is true, as we have related, that we conferred with a spinster who desired AI, but her request was a manifestation of an emotional instability. [W]e believe that any display of interest in this operation by an unmarried woman is indicative of psychological distress . . .[88]

One can only imagine what results the "psychological evaluation" of a lesbian might yield in the office of a physician such as Dr. Finegold, in a state or country where lesbian sexual expression is still criminalized, or where it is still on the books as a mental illness.

Interestingly, in some accounts, lesbians are more likely to pass the psychological screening test than heterosexual women and couples are. During one six-year period at a Connecticut clinic that requires pre-insemination counseling, two heterosexual couples and a married woman who claimed to be single were denied insemination, and three more were told to resolve some personal and couples' issues before returning to inseminate. Not one of the twenty-three lesbian couples that sought insemination was turned away.[89] In a similar finding, unmarried heterosexual women in Belgium are more likely to fail the psychological test than lesbians who are in couples. In one study, sixteen of twenty-one single heterosexual women in Belgium were denied access to AI for psychological reasons, while at the same clinic fourteen out of fifteen requests from lesbians were fulfilled. One can only wonder if, at least in some contexts, relationship stability is becoming seen as more predictive of emotional stability than heterosexuality.[90]

Even with these positive signs, many physicians still deny insemination to lesbians.[91] Regional differences come into play, as do the individual physician's biases.[92] While the dominant discourses of the medical establishment are egregiously heterosexist and discriminatory, the official position does not reflect an absolute consensus among medical practitioners. Individual physicians have a range of perspectives on the insemination of lesbians. These perspectives are difficult to measure, since facilitating insemination of lesbians is of questionable legality in some states, and the appearance of compliance with laws and medical protocols is in the physician's self-interest. Little attention has been given to the study of physician attitudes toward lesbian AI.

Fighting for Access

Physicians as a group have historically believed they have the right to reject potential AI recipients on a variety of bases. In 1987, one in five women who requested insemination was refused, most of them for nonmedical reasons. And in 1988, 63 percent of doctors (who had each inseminated at least four women in the year prior to the survey) stated that they have or would likely reject a request for AI from a lesbian.[93]

Fortunately, they do not always get away with it, as lesbians are gaining legal rights regarding insemination in countries throughout the developed world. A lesbian couple, one member of which was a physician herself, undertook one successful effort in British Columbia. In 1995, Tracy Potter and Sandra Benson took to court the physician who had denied them access to his AI program, Dr. Gerald Korn.[94] Dr. Korn, who had provided insemination services to over a thousand women at the time of the suit and estimated that four or five had been lesbians, argued that his discrimination against them was justifiable since he did not want to be party to legal proceedings should they split. His previous experience was as a witness in a 1984 case of a lesbian couple that split up and fought over support of the children that he had helped them to bear. He said that case had resulted in negative publicity for his practice and calls criticizing him for providing AI services for lesbians. He stopped providing lesbians with AI, but continued to include them in his other OB/GYN practices.

When Dr. Korn denied them AI services, Potter and Benson went into multi-task mode. They procured sperm from California, and the physician of the pair inseminated her partner and filed a complaint against Korn with the College of Physicians and Surgeons of British Columbia. When the College responded that in the absence of emergency or urgent need, Dr. Korn had a right to deny them services, Potter and Benson filed a complaint with the British Columbia Council of Human Rights. They won because of an equal accommodation clause of the British Columbia Human Rights Act. The Council of Human Rights found that physicians are required to comply with the clause prohibiting denial "to any person or class of persons any accommodation, service, or facility customarily available to the public," specifically including discrimination based on family status and sexual orientation. Potter and Benson were awarded CAN $896.44 for the extra expense they incurred obtaining AI elsewhere and CAN $2,500 for emotional injury. Dr. Korn appealed to the British Columbia Supreme Court in 1996, but Potter and Benson won again. The Supreme Court even awarded them costs.

Legal scholar Holly Harlow discusses the widespread discrimination that women without husbands face at the hands of the medical establishment when trying to inseminate. She points out that (married) women began to consult their doctors about AI even before the turn of the twentieth century. The physicians with whom these women consulted were often adamantly opposed to this procedure because they believed that such a proposition came from the devil.[95] It is debatable whether, as we approach the twenty-first century, physicians who refuse to inseminate single women still operate under that premise. While contemporary physicians may or may not share the theological suppositions of their turn-of-the-century counterparts, they continue to abjure and obstruct the insemination of lesbians. Such doctors often cite the belief that unmarried women seeking insemination are emotionally and psychologically imbalanced as their primary reason for denying services.[96]

Although some physicians continue to "hold the line" against lesbian AI, others have changed their practices over the years in the direction of equality for lesbians, sometimes stopping short, however, of equal access. A well-known Boston fertility specialist, who in the past refused to inseminate lesbians, will now inseminate an "unmarried woman"—but only after she undergoes an hour-long "consultation" with a social worker. Conceivably the social worker might not approve the client. Another Boston area medical practice will inseminate almost anyone who walks in the door (at her request), no questions asked about marital status, physical or mental health status, or anything else (except insurance coverage). A large Boston lesbian and gay health center not only orients its AI services toward lesbians but also offers numerous ancillary services—support groups, workshops, and education—to those whom it serves. The exceptional medical providers who offered AI to lesbians before it was popular played a numerically small but important part in the process of normalizing non-nuclear families, often going against the medical protocols of their profession and even possibly breaking the law to do so.

Conclusions

Democratizing access to AI is of the utmost importance for lesbian pro-creative autonomy. Paradoxically, our leading lesbian civil rights organizations have decided not to pursue this issue. According to Kate Kendall, executive director of the National Lesbian Rights Project, enough doctors are willing to inseminate lesbians that, on balance, it is too risky to publicize those who are unwilling. Drawing attention to lesbian insemination has the potential to cause a backlash that results in it being made explicitly illegal.[97] In fact, three states (Hawaii, Minnesota, and Oregon) considered measures to severely curtail or outlaw the insemination of unmarried women in 1995.[98]

Kendall may well be right, in which case I hope this book does not fall into the wrong hands. Still, regardless of when it is undertaken (and that is a serious question), there are several important elements to such a democratizing project. Given that the current system of health care delivery in this country is based on insurance, insurance companies need to take one of two approaches. Either they need to expand their definition of infertile couples to include lesbian couples, so that lesbians will have equal access to insemination and other infertility services. Or, even better, they need to eliminate the category of "infertile couple" altogether, and provide services to any individual, coupled or not, of whatever sexual orientation, who needs and desires them.[99] This latter option more thoroughly enhances the procreative autonomy of women who are not in any kind of couple, which is an important step in the empowerment of women. It would be ironic if the heterosexism of the medical establishment were loosened only to the extent that a woman's partner did not have to be male in order for her to receive fertility benefits. If we support the procreative autonomy of lesbians, then coupledom should not be a prerequisite for any fertility or family-planning related services. Either of these strategies would be an important step in the right direction.

In order for changes in insurance policies to be meaningful, however, access to coverage needs to be universal. Access to humane, appropriate, non-homophobic health care, including infertility services, should be a right, not a privilege. Without such access, changes in coverage will directly affect only the elite who can afford decent insurance.

Medical associations, insurance companies, fertility societies, and individual health care providers ought to come out strongly for motherhood rights for lesbians and other unmarried women. Rather than continuing to strengthen heteropatriarchy, the medical establishment should fight discrimination and the lingering traces of eugenics on all fronts. Anti-homophobic training should be part of every medical education, and a pledge not to discriminate against patients because of sexual orientation should be as mandatory as the Hippocratic oath.

4

Legal Legitimacy and the Lesbian AI "Bastard"

ABSTRACT

Lesbians who seek to inseminate generally face formidable opposition in securing familial protections after the child is born. Every year in the United States, hundreds of lesbian mothers lose custody of their children.[1] While most of these are children conceived through previous heterosexual relationships, lesbian mothers in families started with AI are legally vulnerable in numerous ways. Lesbian AI's potential threat to patriarchal power structures is recognized and reflected in laws that regulate it.

Lesbians using the legal system employ both feudal and modern family discourses to make their cases. Ultimately, however, neither the feudal nor the modern family model is adequate to safeguard the integrity of intentional lesbian families. This is in part because lesbian AI is thoroughly ultramodern, and in part because it challenges the heteropatriarchal foundations of both feudal and modern family models.

Legal Legitimacy and the AI "Bastard"

The law defines what is okay and what is not. Frequently, the law gets to say What Is. Even more than other powerful discourses that decree right and wrong, the law gets to enforce its rules in our lives, to decide who has power.[2] The power of the law renders it an obvious, and crucial, site for subversive interventions. The legal arena is the battleground where emergent family forms fight for their rights to exist.

Just as inseminating lesbians continue to challenge the medical hegemony over AI, they also challenge legal structures that have kept them marginalized and without rights. The intentional lesbian family, along with other "ultramodern" families, is challenging the dominance of hetero-patriarchal family values, and fighting to win.

Three major types of cases relating to lesbian AI have been brought to court. The first is when a sperm donor sues for paternal status and its attendant rights, which range from decision-making power over education and medical care to unsupervised visitation or even custody. The second is when a lesbian couple splits up, and the biological mother uses her legal advantage to deny the non-biological mother parental status or rights. The third is when a lesbian couple uses the legal system in an attempt to gain rights for their family, such as second-parent adoption.

Discerning the frequency of such legal activity is impossible, since many, if not most, such cases are sealed to protect the privacy of family members. Even the National Center for Lesbian Rights (NCLR), the organization at the forefront of the struggle to protect lesbian rights since 1972, has no hard numbers. According to NCLR Executive Director Kate Kendall, less than 10 percent of inseminations result in such lawsuits. In over 90 percent of the cases, individuals resolve problems without recourse to the courts. Sperm donor paternity suits, actions by non-biological co-mothers, and second-parent adoptions are very different types of cases. When viewed together, they bring into sharp relief the legal system's "logic" about the proper behavior of mothers, fathers, and families.

Seemingly contradictory laws and decisions around lesbian AI are tied together by the same sexist logic that undergirds all family law: distrust of independently mothering women, the will to find every child a father, no matter how undesirable,[3] and the condemnation of lesbian relationships.[4] At the same time, the law is fraught with contradictions and competing interests between feudal and modern models of the family. This instability within juridical discourse allows both progressivism and grandstanding on the part of law-making bodies. The simmering contradictions between feudal, modern, and ultramodern family models are brought to a boiling point in the matter of lesbian AI.

The discursive disruptions entailed by lesbian AI confront the law with family structures outside its frame of reference. Along with the more publicized ethical issues to emerge from technologically assisted or contractual procreation, the issues raised by AI regularly end up in court. Frozen embryos, "surrogate" mothers who want out of their contracts, test-tube babies, fetal tissue use by science and industry, and cloning are all matters of legal contention.[5] Possibly the earliest instance of a sperm donor suing for paternal rights is the 1987 New Jersey case known as *C.M. v. C.C.* In this decision, visitation rights were awarded to the donor of semen used at an in-home insemination.[6] Inseminated mothers also have sued their doctors to reveal sperm donors' identities.[7]

Courts have been asked to decide how to define "mother," "father," and "family" when a lesbian has a baby with her female companion as co-parent and without a man. Courts have been charged with resolving philosophical challenges such as: Is a sperm donor a father? Are his parents the child's grandparents? Can a child have two mothers? Who has standing before the court if the mothers split up? Who gets access to whose health insurance, hospital visiting privileges, intestate succession, citizenship, tax deductions, and the host of other privileges accorded "legitimate" family members by law?

In each of these cases, the law has a dilemma. Either it can respond as if the new family forms do not exist, denying them legitimacy and rights, recuperating family members and others back into traditional patriarchal norms (e.g., the co-mother has *no* standing before the court, the sperm donor *is* the father), or it can attempt to transform generations of precedent based in "father right" into something that resembles present realities. In either case, much is at stake as judicial discretion permits idiosyncratic (and widely varying) precedents to be set by individual courts. The legal arena provides a direct window onto the confrontations with state power currently taking place at the boundaries of the family. Lesbian AI is at one leading edge of struggles by mother-headed families to gain cultural legitimacy along with legal rights and protections. Legal rulings use the same underlying cultural resources as do physicians, politicians, and psychoanalysts to justify male power over women and children, as well as over definitions of legal and cultural "legitimacy." Vacillating unevenly between conservatism and utopianism, the law both resists and is a medium for lesbian family empowerment.

As of 2002, all but three U.S. states and the District of Columbia have laws on the books regarding AI.[8] Twenty-eight of these states require "husband's consent" before a woman can be inseminated, which stipulation has been interpreted by the courts as barring the insemination of lesbians and unmarried women. Three states proposed legislation in 1995 that would have outlawed the insemination of unmarried women. Only ten states have equal rights laws that protect the basic civil rights of lesbians and their families from discrimination in areas such as housing, work, and public accommodations.[9] And not one state in the union recognizes lesbian or gay marriage. In fact, as of 2001, thirty-four states had enacted laws specifically banning same-sex marriage.[10] Since same-sex couples are denied the right to legally marry anywhere in the United States, the enactment of laws specifically banning such marriages is beyond gratuitous. It is a political statement of disapproval of lesbian and gay relationships.[11]

Although no state has yet legalized lesbian marriage, Vermont's Civil Union law does provide marriage-like rights to same-sex couples. It applies marriage's rules of adoption as well as child custody and support to these unions. Most importantly for lesbian AI practice, it extends the rights of a married couple to the parties of a civil union with respect to a child of whom either party becomes the natural parent during the union. In other words, the non-biological mom has automatic parental rights and responsibilities toward the biological child of her partner.[12] It is too early to get a sense of the enforceability of these rights, as none of these provisions have been tested through a custody battle, even within Vermont, and other states would not necessarily enforce the civil union provisions if a bio-mom fled the state to renege.[13]

Lesbian AI should not be seen as entirely distinct from lesbian adoption. Adoption is the other major way intentional lesbian families are made, and often AI and adoption go hand in hand, with the non-biological mother seeking to legally adopt the child borne by her partner in a process called "second-parent adoption" or "co-parent adoption." Still, many lesbians embrace AI as a liberating alternative to the often expensive, protracted, and personally intrusive experience of adoption (assuming adoption by lesbians is even legal in a particular country or state). In the United States, only three states specifically forbid or limit adoption by gay and lesbian couples. Florida prohibits adoption by "homosexuals."

Mississippi bans same-sex couples from adopting. Utah "prioritizes married heterosexual couples in the placement of children for foster care and adoption." Arkansas appears to allow adoption by lesbians and gay men, but has a curious administrative rule prohibiting gay men and lesbians from being foster parents.[14] The situation in some states is less clear. The state of Texas does not allow adoption by unmarried couples, will allow unmarried individuals to adopt, and does not inquire about sexual orientation.[15]

NCLR founder and lesbian legal advocate Donna Hitchens developed second-parent adoption (also sometimes called co-parent or step-parent adoption) in the early 1980s to protect lesbian-mother families.[16] In second-parent adoption, a lesbian mother and her partner may apply to have the latter designated as the child's second parent, without relinquishing her own parental status. This differs from the usual process of adoption in the United States, in which any living biological parents must relinquish their parental rights before someone else can adopt the child. If a mother marries a man who wants to adopt her children legally, the children's father must first relinquish his paternal status. Both men cannot be fathers at once. If a person who is not married to either parent wants to adopt the children, both parents must first relinquish their parental status. Therefore, if an inseminating lesbian mother wants her partner to co-adopt their baby, she is legally required to relinquish her own legal parenthood first. In second-parent adoption, this requirement is waived in recognition of the lesbian family unit, so that the child can have the legal and social benefits of a family with two parents. As of 2001, twenty-three U.S. states plus the District of Columbia have granted second-parent adoptions by lesbian co-mothers, either by statute or by court order.[17] In fifteen states, a court has ruled that the state adoption law permits second-parent adoptions by same-sex couples.[18]

Unless and until they are upheld on appeal, those adoptions are still vulnerable to legal challenge.[19] In four states and the District of Columbia, an appellate court has ruled that the state adoption law permits second-parent adoptions by same-sex couples.[20] In these states, the adoptions are safe from legal challenge. In three states, the adoption law explicitly permits second-parent adoption by same-sex couples.[21] In one of these, California, the law specifies that only those same-sex couples registered with the state as domestic partners be allowed second-parent adoption. In four U.S. states, an appellate court has ruled that the state adoption law does not allow for second-parent adoption by same-sex couples.[22]

One of the earliest second-parent adoptions took place in 1992, when a New York court allowed a six-year-old boy's co-mother to adopt him legally, without affecting the parental rights of his biological mother. The mothers, a law professor and a psychologist, had been involved for several years before making the joint decision that one of them would inseminate and that they would equally mother their child. When their son was four years old, they went to court to pursue "second-parent adoption" for the co-mother. They cited the son's pressing need to have his relationship with both parents protected by law.

As reported in the *New York Times*, the court recognized the social-psychological importance of the legal adoption. "There is significant emotional benefit to [the child] from adoption," the court said.[23] "Separate or together, the adoption brings [the child] the additional security conferred by formal recognition in an organized society. As he matures, his connection with two involved, loving parents will not be a relationship seen outside the law." Co-parent adoption has another important benefit as well. In lesbian couples that break up, those co-mothers who had legally adopted their children were more likely to obtain shared custody, and pay child support, than those who didn't legally adopt.[24]

Patricia Williams writes that the law possesses something akin to a life force, and living outside the law can be a kind of death.

> I was [recently] reminded of something I once read in Hans Peter Duerr's book *Dreamtime:* "In archaic times, a person who stood outside the law of a culture was considered dead by ordinary people." . . . I found it riveting, this idea of illegitimacy as a form of death, of legality as its own life force. . . . What is the "law of our culture," I have been asking myself. Who are the "ordinary," real-life people in our society who hold this power of "considered" death? Who are the unreal nonpersons who ghost-walk through the underworld of the illegitimate?[25]

It is this social death, signified by the word for lesbian AI offspring—"illegitimate"—against which intentional lesbian families are fighting, and which second-parent adoption resists. The valorization of intensive mothering and nearly "traditional" family norms used in struggles for second-parent adoption draws significantly on the feudal strain in the discourse of family law.

Legal Status of Lesbianism

Internationally, the legal situation of lesbians is mixed. According to the International Gay and Lesbian Human Rights Commission (IGLHRC), eighty-six countries criminalize sexuality between consenting adults of the same sex.[26] In effect, even being a lesbian in these places is illegal. While some of these laws refer only to gay male sex, the IGLHRC cautions, "Please bear in mind that sodomy laws used to prosecute men have also been used to prosecute women and transsexuals, e.g. in India." Finally, many countries, and several U.S. states, maintain "morality laws" that can be used to intimidate, harass, and arrest lesbians. On the positive side, all sodomy laws in Canada, the countries of the European Union, and the United States have been overturned.

Thirteen U.S. states, plus Puerto Rico, still criminalized lesbian sexual expressions when the U.S. Supreme Court overturned all sodomy laws in 2003.[27] Fines ranged from $500 in South Carolina, Florida, and Texas, to $2,000 in Louisiana. Jail time ranged from sixty days in easygoing Florida to between five years and life in Idaho. Excluding Idaho with its life sentence, the average jail time in U.S. states that banned sodomy was about six years and nine months.

The states and countries in which lesbian sexuality is illegal can be difficult to identify, however, because of the ambiguities of the law applied to lesbian sexual expressions. Legal terms such as "buggery," "sodomy," "penetration," and "unnatural acts" are based on phallocentric premises and therefore rarely specify whether they include lesbian sexuality.

Of course, the overwhelming majority of lesbian sexual activities were never prosecuted by any U.S. state, yet these laws had a chilling effect. As legal scholar Ruthann Robson explains,

> These statutes [that would imprison someone for lesbian sexual expression] are the legal text of lesbian sexuality. Enacted and codified, inter-

preted and applied, these statutes are the legislative pronouncements and judicial interpretations. . . . They are supporting legal text for any feelings any of us might have that our sexuality is wrong.[28]

Almost all U.S. states have codes that at least make reference to alternative insemination. Only Maine, Pennsylvania, South Dakota, and Vermont (plus Puerto Rico and the U.S. Virgin Islands) have no statutory laws that mention human AI. Since not all state law is included in the records available on Lexis-Nexis, it is possible that even these states have some relevant law on the books. The laws of the remaining forty-six states plus the District of Columbia vary widely in comprehensiveness, but they rarely contradict each other.

Laws pertaining to AI fall under many different parts of state codes, including the regulation of potentially HIV-spreading biological material, confidentiality of certain court records, provisions for birth certificates, regulation or prohibition of surrogacy, and mandate or limitation of insurance coverage. But by far the most common concern of the laws is married paternity: affirming the rights and especially the responsibilities of the consenting husband of a married woman who undergoes anonymous donor insemination. Thirty-four states (about 70 percent) have or refer to wording that a consenting husband of a married recipient of donor AI is for purposes of law the child's "natural" and legitimate father.[29] Many states go further, taking particular care to include children through donor insemination by a man's wife in inheritance of his estate and cross-referencing general child support laws to the codes on AI.[30] Far fewer (eighteen) specify that the donor is not the father, perhaps because men try to get out of obligations to children far more than they try to get into them.[31] The statutes in some states seem stereotypical of what we would expect from that state. California's reference ample litigation. Connecticut's are primarily concerned with estates and inheritance. Those of most small states are sparse.

Few laws concerning AI have criminal penalties attached to them. (Exceptions include case law in California where a father through "heterologous" AI was found guilty of criminal non-support, and one in Georgia where a non-physician who performs AI is guilty of a felony.) In general, the criminal penalties are attached to the knowing or negligent use of untested or HIV-positive sperm for artificial insemination. Sixteen states have stipulations related to HIV in their AI-related statutes, including two (Delaware and Iowa) for which that is the only area of AI regulated by law.[32] In addition to six states that limit the practice of artificial insemination to physicians and those supervised by them, ten state codes only address AI performed by a licensed physician.[33] Interestingly, four states offer the possibility of an inseminating mother agreeing in advance that her "heterologous" sperm donor (not her husband) would have rights. Only five states have references to case law involving lesbians.[34] Most cases involve nonbiological mothers seeking visitation, but one involves a biological mom seeking and winning child support. Another involved a case of a woman impersonating a man, including signing the consent forms as the inseminating mother's husband, and then being ordered to pay parental support.

Since the situation of the intentional lesbian family is not specified in the legal codes of any state, courts are at liberty to apply existing laws about lesbians (if any), and about AI (if any), as they go along.[35] This excess of judicial discretion leads to an extreme lack of consistency. Not only do states vary widely, but also individual courts draw erratically (though with predictably sexist and heterosexist results) from family, contract, and adoption law to make their decisions.[36] Thus, parental rights frequently granted to nonbiological parents such as grandparents and stepparents are often denied to lesbian co-mothers.[37] Co-mothers and their nonbiological children enjoy no familial standing vis-à-vis each other, and hence no legal protection ordinarily granted to parents and children in the literally hundreds of laws that bear on families in areas such as housing, immigration, Social Security, insurance, child support and visitation, and intestate succession.[38] As with many aspects of the relationship between lesbians and the law, it is impossible to know how many such cases have come before the courts, or how they have been decided, since most are not public record and many have been sealed.

Even the biological mother's biological and legal ties to her children are not always enough to sustain her custody when a "third party" such as her parents wants to take it from her. Several high-profile cases, as well as innumerable unremarked ones, involve lesbians who lost custody of their children to their parents (the children's grandparents), based solely, or primarily, on lesbianism.[39]

It is possible, however, to have a more sanguine perspective. Legal scholar Nan Hunter, for instance, puts a positive gloss on the current state of lesbian family law:

> The law's changes to protect sexual dissent within the family will occur at different speeds in different places, which might not be so bad. Family law has always been a province primarily of state rather than federal regulation, and often has varied from state to state; grounds for divorce, for example, used to differ dramatically depending on geography. What seems likely to occur in the next wave of family cases is the same kind of variability in the legal definition of the family itself. Those very discrepancies may help to denaturalize concepts like "marriage" and "parent," and to expose the utter contingency of the sexual conventions that, in part, construct the family.[40]

While I do not share Hunter's optimistic long view, it bears mentioning since it offers a glimmer of hope in an otherwise somewhat dismal state of affairs.

Even if this long view turns out to be correct, lesbians using AI today remain extremely vulnerable to paternity claims by sperm donors. This legal vulnerability leaves many lesbians with anonymous sperm donation as the only option for creating families free from the threat of paternity challenges. However, legally sanctioned discrimination against lesbians by doctors, sperm banks, and insurance companies makes access to these services fraught with obstacles.[41] Thus, both medical power and lesbians' low legal status are reinforced.

The inability or unwillingness of the courts to recognize and protect lesbian families is not only a matter of homophobia. It is also a matter of how the legal family is defined.[42] It is instructive to look at the legal position of men who are in an analogous situation to lesbian co-mothers. They may be so invisible that there is no name to describe them, but they play a crucial role in the sustenance of many heterosexual-parent families. These are men who, in differing degrees, care for and support mothers through pregnancy, birth, and childrearing. Men who partner mothers "can be valuable for the strong, mutual, irrational, and emotional attachments they form with children and for the love and respite they give to mothers."[43] The court is not kind to them. Heterosexual men who fall outside the legal definition of the family are frequently excluded from parental standing and rights. A man that marries or partners with a woman who is pregnant (not with his sperm), cares for her throughout her pregnancy, helps her through labor and birth, and lives with her and the child as the husband/father for a number of years, is likely to be denied parental standing by the court.[44] But a man whose only relationship with a mother was an occasion of PIVMO that led to pregnancy, and who has never previously given the child the time of day, may well have legal standing as a father.[45] If nonbiological social fathers are disempowered by law, it is no surprise that lesbian co-mothers are even more so. Barbara Bennett Woodhouse argues that men who develop nonbiolegal familial relationships with children and their mothers are treated by the courts as if they are "generous fools" and denied legal standing as fathers. Conversely, men who "get something for nothing" by impregnating a woman and disappearing, are rewarded by the courts with parental standing. Lesbian co-mothers, I would argue, are also frequently viewed as "generous fools" not only by the courts but also in their communities.

The failure to see the nonbiological mother as a "real" parent is grounded not only in homophobia but also in racist and class-based patriarchal traditions. These traditions define fatherhood legally while discounting the actual nurturing and commitment that arguably should define familial relationships. Further, the more socially marginalized the co-mother is, the less seriously her claim as a "real" parent is taken. First, co-mothers are neither biogenetically nor legally related to their spouses and children. Second, since care work is invisible and devalued in our society, so is the care work performed by the co-mother. Third, family is defined in racialized and class-based terms, so that people of color and low-income people are not seen as having "real" families worthy of protections and rights. Most co-mothers are low-income and/or of color, and so are even less likely than white, liquid-class co-mothers to have their family status acknowledged and honored. Finally, heteronormativity leads to the perception that lesbian families do not, and should not, exist.

Lesbians suffer legally sanctioned oppression in virtually all sectors of their lives, including against their families.[46] Anti-lesbian discrimination in areas such as housing, employment, marriage, taxation, intestate succession, and immigration are conjoined with anti-lesbian harassment, assault (up to and including murder), police indifference to or participation in such crimes, and the criminalization of lesbian sexual expression. Lesbians (and other women who do not conform to the gender and sexual norms of their cultures) across the globe suffer severe, often legally sanctioned punishment, which include rulings depriving them of dependent children. In a project documenting lesbian human rights in thirty countries, National Center for Lesbian Rights (NCLR) staff attorney and author of the U.S. report Shannon Minter writes,

> Although the U.S. Supreme Court has recognized that "the rights attached to parenthood are among the 'basic civil rights,'" state courts routinely view lesbians and gay parents as undeserving of the rights afforded to other parents. As a result, the estimated six to fourteen million children with a lesbian or gay parent have little protection against judicial decisions that arbitrarily dissolve or disrupt their families.[47]

She goes on to cite examples of the way that the notions of lesbians as undeserving have played out in child custody and visitation fights:

> Most state courts . . . either deem lesbian and gay parents per se unfit to raise children or deny normal custody and visitation rights based on unfounded bias and stereotypes about lesbian parents. . . . In a highly publicized case in 1994, a Virginia trial court removed Sharon Bottoms' two-year-old son from her custody based solely on the judge's belief that Sharon Bottoms' lesbianism was "immoral" and "illegal." In April 1995, the Virginia State Supreme Court upheld this ruling.[48]

Internationally, the situation is better in some places, and worse in others. According to the International Gay and Lesbian Human Rights Commission, gays and lesbians are excluded everywhere from at least some of the rights and privileges associated with marriage.[49] Despite lesbian and gay legal gains, differences remain between the official treatment of same-sex unions and different-sex marriage.

The Canadian Province of Quebec has progressive laws regarding lesbian families and AI. Although Quebec's Bill 84, "an Act instituting civil unions and establishing new rules of filiation," effective 2002, does not affect marriage in Canada, which is federal, it does create a second legal status—civil union—available to both same-sex and different-sex couples in Quebec with the same rights and responsibilities as marriage. The thousands of changes to the civil code to make this civil union option available are testimony to the wide-reaching rights and obligations associated with marriage. An extensive sub-chapter of the law addresses "filiation of children born of assisted procreation." The filiation is established at birth "between the child, the woman who gave birth to the child and, where applicable, the other party to the parental project."[50] That filiation creates the same rights and obligation as filiation by blood. The child of one member of the union is presumed to be his or her partner's child as well, and that presumption can be rebutted.[51] Importantly, the contributor of genetic material may *not* claim any filiation with the child born of assisted reproduction.[52]

This is exactly the direction I believe the law ought to go. If the registered partner of a lesbian mom who conceived with AI wants to claim that she is not a co-parent, she has the option to do that in court. The assumption, however, is that she is an equal parent with the biological mother, with all of the rights and responsibilities that go along with that status. At the same time, the sperm donor is explicitly banned from claiming paternity, thus protecting the lesbian family's integrity. However, the law has a medicalized notion of lesbians' babies. Unassisted procreation is grounds for a partner to rebut the presumed filiation. And an unmedically produced child may claim filiation with the contributor of the genetic material, with caveats.[53] Finally, the Quebec law has a lesbian-friendly section about the effects of divorce on children. "The dissolution of a civil union does not deprive the children of the advantages secured to them by law or by the civil union contract. The rights and obligations of parents towards their children are unaffected by the dissolution of the union."[54]

Northern European countries began opening marriage with explicit exception of rights related to children. Denmark's 1989 law became a model for many (Iceland, Norway, and Sweden) including rights of property, inheritance, immigration, taxation, and social security. However, the original law, and those based on it, stipulated that same-sex partners could only adopt children biologically related to their partner (also known as second-parent adoption). Such discrimination was upheld in 1998 by the Danish parliament, which voted to maintain the ban on unmarried women, including lesbians, receiving AI. Since then, Denmark, Iceland, and most recently Sweden have extended adoption rights to gays and lesbians. France's domestic partnership excludes adoption rights. French lesbian couples also do not have a legal right to AI. Some provinces extend more rights than their national governments do, including Catalonia (Spain), but again without adoption rights.

The Netherlands is the most comprehensive in its recognition of lesbian and gay marriage, having moved to almost complete parity of same-sex marriages.[55] Marriage was opened to lesbians and gay men in 2001, but with three distinctions all related to descent: non-biological parents had to adopt the children born to their partners, international adoption was not available, and their children could not become king or queen. The first of those distinctions was mitigated as of 1 January 2002. Now, non-biological parents have an equal share of the parental authority and maintenance duties toward the children of their partners. However, if they want full parental status, they have to go through an adoption procedure. Gays and lesbians continue to lack access to international adoption, however, and their children continue to be denied ascension to the throne.

Feminist Legal Reform

Feminists have had mixed success in seeking social justice through legal reform. The law has a progressive, utopian aspect that makes it a natural site of struggles for social justice, and feminists have successfully exploited this element of the law to substantially eliminate statutes that deny equality to women. These include both positive protections (e.g., the right to vote, the right to equal education, the right to hold property) and prohibitions against anti-woman discrimination (e.g., maternity-leave laws, anti-sexual harassment laws). The law, however, also has a profoundly conservative aspect that is unresponsive to many elements of a feminist social justice agenda. Feminist legal scholars who confront the intransigence of legally codified androcentrism may come away pessimistic about the law as an instrument for social change. As feminist legal theorists Martha Fineman and Nancy Sweet Thomadsen write,

> When the goals and insights of feminism contend with powerfully entrenched legal institutions feminist ideals seem inevitably to become

distorted and co-opted, while the law remains essentially unchanged. Although particular or partial legal changes may occur, these "victories" often lay the ground for doctrines that harm rather than help women.[56]

The intransigence of legal patriarchy leads at times to despair and even to "exit" from the legal arena.[57] Fortunately, feminists and lesbians in the legal field, as elsewhere, fight burnout and usually rise again to continue the good fight.

While specific laws and the law in general claim to be neutral, objective, and "fair," they are widely criticized by feminists as serving the interests of the powerful. Local, state, and federal laws that pertain to lesbian AI seem incoherent, disjointed, and even random at first glance. But recurring themes in the narratives of appellants, defendants, and jurists reveal a pattern that subtends most of the decisions in this matter. In trials, and especially in judicial decisions, we can observe the segments of judicial narratives that are frozen into the discrete "rules" that, together, comprise the law. Individual laws are seen as frozen moments in the stream of larger, usually unarticulated, narratives.[58] These narratives derive from ideologically dominant discourses and have the invisibility of "common sense." In such assessments, the law is exposed as ideologically interested, fundamentally biased, and therefore unjust.

Anthropologist Clifford Geertz spoke about common sense as that which seems obvious but which is actually culturally constructed. He used examples from diverse cultures, allowing readers to recognize that what is "common sense" elsewhere can be non-obvious or even untrue in Western culture. Calling something "common sense" is usually a conservative appeal to an unreflective normality. As critical theorists, we look for the historical underpinnings and the political implications of discourses that we construe as common sense.

Many have criticized the law as constraining to feminist perspectives due to its fetishistic devotion to rationality and positivism.

> Law . . . insists upon arguments it deems rational and coherent rather than ambiguous or contradictory. As feminists in diverse disciplines have shown, standards of what is rational reflect the interests of those who currently hold power, whose authority is affirmed by how neutral and inevitable these standards appear to be . . . Likewise, courts prefer re-

ductive, dichotomous legal categories to overlapping or ambiguous ones; consequently, a black woman claiming discrimination because of the combination of her race and sex may be unable to fit her claim to the law's narrow requirements of either race or sex discrimination.[59]

This line of critique also extends to family law.[60] The sexual conservatism of U.S. law is of course built on a legacy of patriarchy, slavery, and genocide, in which double-talk and abstraction were used to uphold (profitably) unjust institutions such as chattel slavery.[61] Obfuscation and abstraction ("legal reasoning") are inseparable from U.S. legal history, as such rhetorical strategies were necessitated by the evils to be justified. Further, the reliance of the courts on precedents forecloses the possibilities for more than reformist changes in the law. Writing of the ways in which law as an institution has "both helped to implement and constrained feminist agendas," feminist legal scholars Bartlett and Kennedy identify the concept of precedent as a conservative constraint.

> One such constraint is the law's respect for precedent. Law may be changed, but because law purports to preserve institutional stability and continuity, reform must build from existing legal precedents and doctrines. For feminists, this requirement presents two problems. First, existing precedents are often decidedly androcentric, taking for granted and reinforcing a status quo that is more favorable to male interests than to female ones. Second, arguments that deviate significantly from precedent or accepted doctrine are often considered extreme and thus are less likely to be successful than moderate proposals.[62]

Legal actions regarding AI suffer directly from this adherence to precedent. The inability of courts to recognize family forms outside of their historical framework disadvantages those who seek to have lesbian families protected. If, as literary scholars Janice Doane and Devon Hodges argue, nostalgia is not only a feeling but also a rhetorical strategy, then the law is a nostalgic discourse extraordinaire.[63]

This is precisely the rhetorical strategy used in legal texts (statutes, rulings) as well as by those who resist expanding the boundaries of the ("legitimate") family to include lesbians and their children. Through reliance on precedent, the law is able to all but deny the realities of family diversity. Through a continual reference to the heteropatriarchal family norm, legal doctrine enshrines that family form at the expense of all others. As legal scholars Carl Stychin and Didi Herman wrote, "The conservatism of the legal establishment should never be underestimated."[64]

Today, unjust individual laws are still supported ideologically by oppressive narratives. Bias against lesbians in custody rulings can be vague. Unless the perpetrator is explicit about his or her anti–lesbianism, the victim may be left wondering if she was mistreated because she is a woman, because she is a lesbian, or for other reasons entirely. In some cases, it may be easier to cope with and fight explicit heterosexism than veiled heterosexism in which the victim can never prove discrimination. Discussing the material and psychological violence of such silence, international human rights activist Rachel Rosenbloom writes,

> Not only do most violations of lesbians' human rights (like violations
> of women's rights more generally) take place within the "private"
> sphere, but the silence that surrounds lesbianism adds an additional layer
> of difficulty in documenting such violations. . . . The rules may be
> unwritten—or even unspoken—but they are very real, and the official
> silence surrounding lesbianism does not make the prohibition of it any
> less powerful; it only makes it harder to document, respond to, or resist
> the abuses that lesbians experience.[65]

Legal practices and discourses strongly support the patriarchal family. Most states protect the privacy of all parties involved in the insemination of a married woman, as long as she has her husband's consent.[66] The law typically protects the married couple from intrusion by the sperm donor. The husband is listed as the child's father on the birth certificate. The law also protects the sperm donor from any legal claims by the child or the child's mother. By institutionalizing these protections, the law supports such arrangements, extends legitimacy to the offspring and sanctions them socially.[67]

The law does not bestow the same protections on lesbian mothers who use AI. In fact, it could be argued that the law encodes its disapproval. As legal scholar Martha Minow has noted, when legal rules bear so little relation to how actual people live their lives, the law is merely codified ideology: a statement of what lawmakers do and do not endorse.[68] For lesbians, as for other unmarried women, their sperm donors' parental rights may be contingent on the participation of a physician in the insemination, thereby making the women who inseminate without a doctor doubly vulnerable to intrusion by the sperm donor.[69] Because unmarried women's legal protection (from paternity claims) is often limited to those cases of AI assisted by a physician, doctors who refuse to inseminate single or lesbian women add to the legally precarious position such women already occupy. According to editors of the Harvard Law Review, "By making the donor's legal status hinge on a doctor's participation, these statutes give the medical profession an unjustifiable power to determine who will and will not have access to AI without the threat of paternity claims."[70] Since no "presumptive father" (husband) exists who could invalidate a sperm donor's paternity claims, lesbians are denied explicit legal protection from such claims.[71]

The early California case of *Jhordan C. v. Mary K.* illustrates this problem. In 1978, a lesbian couple, Mary and Victoria, agreed to inseminate Mary with the sperm of Jhordan, a man they knew. They agreed that he would see the baby only once when the baby was born, with no further contact. After the birth, Jhordan began to demand more involvement in the baby's—and hence the mothers'—life. The mothers let him visit approximately once a month for the first five months, and then terminated visitation, asserting that they had never agreed to it in the first place. In 1980, Jhordan took Mary to court, filing a paternity action. In June 1982, he was declared the legal father, was granted weekly visitation with the child in Mary's home, and was ordered to pay monthly child support. The reason cited by the court was that Mary had not been inseminated under the supervision of a physician. Her sperm donor's paternal rights had not been extinguished, and she was unprotected from paternity claims.[72] Thus, the courts upheld medical hegemony over AI, and punished a lesbian mother who dared to inseminate outside of its control.

Lesbian co-mothers typically must meet higher standards than other nonbiological parents in order to be recognized legally as parents. The legal standing frequently granted to adoptive parents, grandparents, and step-parents due to their status as de facto parents, people standing *in loco parentis*, functional parents, or psychological parents is typically denied to lesbian co-parents.[73] In one study, sociologist Cameron L. Macdonald compares custody disputes in three cases, two involving "surrogate motherhood" (one of which involves "gestational surrogacy") and one involving AI.[74] Macdonald shows that, in each case, the women are held to a higher standard of "bonding" with the child than the men are, and further, that no amount of "bonding" with the child is enough to give a lesbian co-mother parental standing before the court.

The definition of the family used by courts deciding cases involving AI discriminates against lesbian families. The legal or "formal" definition of the family denies the parenthood of the co-mother regardless of her actual emotional and material daily relationship to the child and to his or her biological mother. Such a definition typically allows only people related by biology, adoption, or marriage to be legally recognized as family. Under this legal definition, lesbian co-mothers have less legal standing, despite years of involvement in raising their (nonbiological) child(ren), than the sperm donor who has never met the child(ren). The nonbiological mother is therefore denied legal parental rights—housing, immigration, welfare, insurance, custody/visitation, intestate succession—as well as freed legally from her parental responsibilities.[75]

Feminist legal scholars and practicing attorneys alike have made the case for an alternative "functional" definition of the family to take the place of the current formal one. According to the American Civil Liberties Union (ACLU) definition, a "functional" parent:

1. Will have spent considerable time with the child at some point in the child's life, typically by living with the child for some significant period(s) of time;
2. Will have for significant periods of time been responsible for, and called upon, to make day-to-day decisions in the child's existence;
3. Will have played a significant role in the broader decisions about a child's upbringing (such as . . . school, . . . religion, . . . medical care . . ., etc.);
4. Will have come to play this de facto parental role with the consent of the existing parent or parents who have legal custody of the child.[76]

The ACLU also argues for consideration of whether the child considers the person in question a parent figure and of the child's wishes (without discounting the child's maturity).[77]

One illustration of the problems caused by a rigid "formal" definition of the family is the New York case of *Alison D. v. Virginia M.* Alison and Virginia lived together for several years as a lesbian couple, and decided to start a family together, with Virginia inseminating and Alison providing the sole economic support. When the baby was three years old, the couple split up. Alison continued to provide economic support and had weekly overnight visitation with the child. The child also maintained close contact with Alison's parents, whom he knew as his grandparents. After two years, Virginia started to limit Alison's contact with the child. When Virginia attempted to cut off all contact between Alison and the child, Alison took her to court for continued visitation (not custody). The court declined to hear her case, stating that as a "non-parent" she had no standing before the court. Remarkably, the court added, "a child cannot have two mothers."[78]

Fortunately, not all courts share this court's adherence to a hetero-nuclear definition of family. In the United States, there have been many successes among lesbian couples seeking to have both parents legally recognized as such. As discussed earlier, second-parent adoption is available in a small number of U.S. jurisdictions, and will probably become available in more. Also, lesbians not using AI have been able in some instances to have both of their names listed on the birth certificate of a child adopted by both of them. In several countries, it is possible to have two women recognized as a child's legal parents.

Israel's High Court of Justice, its highest court, faced the question of whether a child can have two mothers nearly twenty years after the New York court, but reached the opposite conclusion. A lesbian couple, Ruthie and Nicole Berner-Kadish were joint U.S.-Israeli citizens and co-parents of their young son, whom Ruthie had given birth to and Nicole had legally adopted in the United States. When they went to Israel and attempted to register their son as an Israeli citizen, however, the Ministry of the Interior refused to acknowledge that the child had two mothers, asserting that the listing of two women on the birth certificate was a "mistake" since "everyone knows a child cannot have two mothers." Therefore he would only register the biological mother on his Israeli citizenship papers. The mothers took the case to Israel's High Court of Justice, where they found a more progressive judge. This judge explained in his ruling that many children have both a mother and a stepmother, and many others have both a birth mother and an adoptive mother, so as a matter of "fact," the listing of the second mother on the official papers was not a "mistake." This was an important case not only for the family involved but also for future cases involving same-sex parents in Israel.[79]

In both cases, the courts, under the cover of legal neutrality, made rulings with powerful political implications. The Israeli court found, as a matter of "fact," that no error had been made in the assertion that a child has two mothers. The New York court, by contrast, dealt a devastating blow to Alison, her son, and his grandparents, and used its discursive and institutional power to de-legitimize intentional lesbian families. The latter discursive move may be seen as part of the propagandistic project described by anthropologist Anna Tsing in "Monster Stories," in which social institutions perpetuate and enforce the categories of anti-mother and anti-family for purposes of social control.[80] This "bastardizing" juridical move has a history as long as the law itself, and is as much about supporting class inequalities (through patrilineage) as it is about racial, gender, and sexual hierarchies.

The law, like medicine, is a mighty discourse. It has the power to socially "legitimate" children, relationships, and families. Legal scholar Patricia Williams' discussions of legitimacy and illegitimacy are extremely apropos of the intentional lesbian family. Discussing the contemporary right wing's efforts to dismantle the welfare state, Williams writes,

> The war on illegitimacy is, to restate the obvious, a way of drawing lines between children who are thought legitimate and those who are not. In terms of its civic consequences, it builds a barrier between legal and illegal children, between those who are all in the family and those who are deemed alien.[81]

She then poses a crucial question:

> But what would happen if all these ["illegitimate"] children were assumed to be "legitimate" . . .? What possibilities could be imagined if

this [welfare] debate were about people the civic circle deemed worthy and deserving?[82]

What indeed? And what would happen if the children of lesbians and their families were assumed to be "legitimate"?

Feudal, Modern, and Postmodern Family Law

Tensions among pre-modern, modern, and postmodern versions of the family are rife within legal discourse and are played out in rulings on lesbian AI. While pre-modern and modern family discourses often cohere so neatly as to be indistinguishable, points of tension within the law have been used as wedges for gaining rights for lesbian family members, as well as in the service of heterosexism and conservatism.

Those seeking to establish rights for intentional lesbian families have utilized both feudal and modern legal strategies. Mothers engaged in custody battles against sperm donors usually draw on modern family discourse to emphasize how sperm donor intrusion violates their rights, previous contracts, and family autonomy. These arguments emphasize the modern definition of family as a binding contract between rational actors who are legally and morally bound to honor their agreements. Lesbian mothers who began their families with AI also employ modern legal discourse in their understanding of the donor as a role explicitly open to negotiation. That individuals are free to choose and define their significant relationships based on individual preferences is at the heart of modern family ideology.[83]

While it might seem at first glance that intentional lesbian families would gain nothing by turning to legal strategies based on feudal family discourses, in fact some lesbian mothers have done just that. One of the chief characteristics of feudal family discourse is the naturalization of family roles, dynamics, and hierarchies. While all cultures have the tendency to draw on "the natural" as a discourse of legitimation and cultural coherence, "the natural" has a special place in Western metaphysics. Particularly in relation to sexuality, medical, legal, religious, and scientific discourses have used "the natural" as a stand-in for what is morally right. For instance, in modern patriarchal discourses, the woman who wanted to have a career, to write, or even to vote, was condemned as morally and medically harmful. Serious doubts were raised as to whether her uterus could survive such "unnatural" activities.[84]

Despite the strength of the association between deviance and the unnatural, paradoxes and contradictions within the discourse are numerous. Literary scholar Eve Kosofsky Sedgwick summarizes the issues by noting a tautology in the description of homosexuality (here referred to as "depravity") as unnatural.

> "A depravity according to nature," like "natural depravity," might denote something that is depraved when measured against the external standard of nature—that is, something whose depravity is unnatural. Either of the same two phrases might also denote, however, something whose proper nature it is to be depraved—that is, something whose depravity is natural. So all the definition accomplishes here is to carry the damning ethical sanctions already accumulated into a new semantic field, that of nature and the *contra naturam*—a field already entangled for centuries with proto-forms of the struggles around homosexual definition.[85]

Still, in relation to sexuality, "the natural" continues to be used for social control. Under modern medical discourse, eroticism between members of the same sex was considered not only deviant, but also unnatural: It both went against the natural order and signified the dissolution of that order. Aspects of women's sexuality that did not fit the constraints of modernist patriarchal ideology—such as clitoral orgasm and lesbian desires—were pathologized as "unnatural." Modernist discourse even joins the divinely sanctioned with "the natural," so that "sins" such as homosexuality and masturbation are considered counter to both God and nature. The law chimes in as enforcing arbiter of right and wrong, deeming certain forms of sexuality legal and others illegal.

Lesbians have long been placed on the wrong side of the "natural"/ "unnatural" tracks by organized religion, medicine, and the law.[86] Even in the twenty-first century, the word "unnatural" comes up in relation to gay and lesbian relationships in legal arguments and judgments (as well as in the proclamations of religious and media pundits). In part due to the legacies of European colonialism, characterization of same-sex eroticism as "unnatural" is not limited to the West.[87] As the International Gay and Lesbian Human Rights Commission reports, "many laws, such as section

377 of the Indian Penal Code, prohibit 'acts against nature,' a term which specifies neither gender nor sexual orientation; however, in practice these laws have generally been enforced only against male homosexual acts."[88] "The family," on the other hand, is seen as the epitome of "naturalness": timeless, sacred, normal, and good. In such narratives, "the family" of course refers only to a narrow set of kinship and gender relations. As Judith Stacey writes, in the United States this designation refers to "the family form that most Americans now consider traditional—an intact nuclear unit inhabited by a male breadwinner, his full-time homemaker wife, and their dependent children."[89]

Lesbians have sought to destigmatize their existence and their families by attaching themselves to the "natural" side of the good-evil divide. Using numerous discursive and practical strategies, lesbians have reasserted the "naturalness" of their lives, often with some success. Lesbians and gay men often find it helpful to articulate themselves as members of a minority group that they are part of through no choice of their own. For many lesbians, this is more than a rhetorical or political strategy. It is the way they experience their lives. It has also been shown that heterosexuals who believe lesbians and gay men have no control over their sexual orientation ("born that way") are more positive and accepting toward them.[90]

This approach to social change has been described as "homophile" in opposition to more supposedly radical "queer" designations, which imply the refusal to assimilate into the plus side of this zero-sum equation. Homophile politics emphasize that gay people are "just like" heterosexuals, normal and wholesome in every way. Lesbian mothers almost always rely on this rhetorical strategy when defending themselves as mothers in custody battles. Lesbians have used such homophile rhetoric, with some success, in the struggle for second-parent adoption.

Ultimately, however, neither the feudal nor the modern family model is adequate to safeguard the integrity of intentional lesbian families or family members.[91] While determined lesbian (biological and nonbiological) mothers have extracted some justice from feudal family discourse, it is overwhelmingly hostile to lesbians. The patriarchal imperative of feudal family ideology is explicit, and includes the judicial desire to "find the child a father" at all costs. Its tenets include failure to recognize "alternative" family forms, legal empowerment of biological fathers at the expense of (all) mothers, and denial of co-mothers' parental status. The explicitly patriarchal presumptions of the feudal strain in family law render it most clearly detrimental to intentional lesbian families.

Modern family discourse has been more hospitable to intentional lesbian families under the law. Yet it too is built on a bedrock of hetero-patriarchal assumptions and fails to protect intentional lesbian families and family members in fundamental regards. Modern family doctrine is bad for AI families in many of the same ways that it is bad for other families. Some of the more egregious abuses structured into the ascendance of modern capitalist values—radical individualism, devaluation of care work, entrenchment and replication of racial, class, and other hierarchies—all contribute to a legal system inadequate, if not inimical, to the interests of most intentional lesbian family members. Because intentional lesbian families are definitively ultramodern and mother-centered, only legal discourses that are also ultramodern and at least somewhat mother-centered might be adequate to their needs for rights, justice, and legitimacy.

5

The Economics of Lesbian Insemination

ABSTRACT

Race and economics are as important as sexuality and gender to understanding lesbian AI. In the United States, lesbian AI (though not lesbian
parenting) is primarily a phenomenon of white, middle- and upper-class
lesbians. This chapter focuses on the commercialization and class-based
stratification of lesbian AI and analyzes their possible causes. It also in-
vestigates the contradictory implications—both alienating and liberating—
for lesbians of buying sperm, particularly from sperm banks.

Stratified Reproduction

All the studies I am aware of show that AI is most frequently practiced by
those with higher incomes.[1] One major study found that 58 percent of the
intentional lesbian families studied had annual household incomes of over
$60,000.[2] In another study, which included both lesbians and heterosexuals,
the only working class people in the entire study were lesbians who self-
inseminated with known sperm donors.[3]

The National Survey of Family Growth (NSFG) is useful here.[4] Data
from this comprehensive survey do not distinguish between AI and other
forms of ART, but the numbers do shed light on access to reproductive
services in the United States. Infertility services in general, and ART in
particular, are stratified along lines of marital status, race, income, and
education, as well as sexual orientation.

First, we see this stratification in the gaps between the numbers of women who consult a fertility specialist and those who end up getting some form of ART. As we might expect, childless married women are by far the most likely to seek and to receive infertility services. Over 20 percent of U.S. married childless women have received any infertility services as compared to just over 2 percent of unmarried childless women. As the level of infertility services becomes more extensive, the disparity between married and unmarried childless women becomes even greater.[5] Married childless women are almost five times as likely as unmarried childless women to have their initial infertility appointment lead to them receiving some form of ART. Perhaps needless to say, lesbians fall under the unmarried category here.

The differences between the treatment of married and unmarried women who have had one or more births were less striking, but remain significant: While married women are just one and one-half times more likely to receive infertility services, they are more than twice as likely to receive ART.[6]

By education, differences can be found not so much in who seeks infertility treatment, but in who receives ART. Fifteen percent of women without a high school diploma have sought treatment, while about 20 percent of women with at least a high school diploma (or GED) have done so.[7] Yet those with a bachelor's degree or higher are twice as likely to receive ART than those with either high school education or only some college, and eleven times as likely to receive ART than women without a high school diploma (or GED).[8]

Poverty-level income is a strong indicator that a woman will not receive ART. While 14.2 percent of women whose income is below the poverty level receive "any services," only 0.1 percent of those women receive ART. In contrast, 20.3 percent of women whose incomes are three times the poverty level receive "any services," and 2.2 percent of them receive ART. So while the wealthiest women are only a bit more likely to seek infertility services than those in poverty, high-income women are twenty-two times as likely to receive ART.[9]

Racial disparities among women receiving ART are also much greater than the disparities in infertility services in general. Whites (non-Hispanic) are only about 25 percent more likely than Hispanics and Blacks to receive any services, yet they are twice as likely as Hispanics and four times as likely as Blacks to receive ART. "Non-Hispanic others," a group we may assume includes many Asian-Americans, are the most likely to receive some form of ART, though the least likely to receive any services.

While this data does not tell us who, or how many people are inseminating, it does provide a picture of how contractual and technological procreation is stratified in the United States. In every case noted above, those with higher social status are more likely to receive ART. It is safe to assume that, at least for those pursuing medical AI, insemination is probably similarly stratified among lesbians. Lesbians who are well above the poverty level, lesbians designated "non–Hispanic white" or "non-Hispanic other," and lesbians with at least a high school diploma (or GED) are likely to inseminate more frequently than other groups of lesbians. As I have discussed, however, it is difficult to get a handle on the demographics of lesbian AI. Low-income women may well inseminate more often than the current research suggests.[10]

Social Class and "Doing Family"

Today's methods of doing AI are expensive, with most of the costs paid to doctors, sperm banks, and lawyers.[11] Even if they use a known sperm donor, most women will want to have him screened for sexually transmissible infections. In the United States, this costs money. To benefit from those unusual cases where the costs of AI are covered by health insurance, you have to be affluent enough to be well insured. If achieving pregnancy is delayed, then a host of (expensive) medical interventions come up for consideration. Buying semen from a sperm bank is expensive as well, with each added enhancement (e.g., a "yes" sperm donor who is willing to be known to the child when she or he turns 18, sperm ready for intrauterine insemination) adding to the cost.

Physicians use their discretion in finding sperm sources. Some are more expensive than others. Women whose physicians buy from sperm banks pay at least the cost of the sperm for each insemination, and often undergo numerous cycles of insemination with frozen and thawed semen before either achieving a pregnancy or giving up. I gathered the following numbers from three sperm banks known to serve the lesbian community, the sperm banks used by Boston's Fenway Community Health Center (a lesbian and gay health center with a large AI program), and the large sperm banks listed on the first page of a Google internet search.[12]

Medical AI typically costs about $500 to $1,000 for the first cycle, and about $300 to $700 for each cycle thereafter.[13] These numbers include the following basic costs:

> Registration at a sperm bank or clinic ($150)
> Health tests ($0–$600)
> Frozen semen ($135–$265 per vial)
> Ovulation-predictor kits ($45–$60)
> Intrauterine insemination ($150–$275; does not include the sperm sample)
> Intracervical insemination ($100 and up; does not include the sperm sample)
> Shipping ($100–$200)

The cost rises with each "enhancement" such as:

> Recipient/donor photo matching ($25–$45)
> Donor audio interview ($25–$35)
> Donor baby photo ($5–$25)
> Donor medical profile: ($10–$15)
> "Doctorate sperm" (donor has, or is in the process of earning, an M.D., Ph.D., J.D., or other doctorate degree) ($280–$335 per vial)
> Sex pre-selection[14] ($475–$3,950)
> Expedited shipping (of sperm, dry ice, liquid nitrogen tank) ($10–$90)
> Weekend appointments (an additional $25–100)
> Counseling of various kinds (e.g., genetic counseling, donor selection counseling, intake counseling) ($60–$600).

While AI is still the least expensive form of technological or contractual procreation, its costs are high enough to keep it out of reach for many. Market forces and class privilege often trump "moral" prohibitions and protocols. Lesbians with cash more easily can find a way to bypass legal, physician, or insurance company proscriptions and inseminate under private medical supervision, while non-wealthy lesbians must shoulder the legal and medical, and therefore psychological, insecurity of self-insemination.

Lesbians inseminating outside of the medical system are aware of the risks of HIV infection. A British study found lesbians inseminating with fresh sperm taking both precautions and risks.[15] On the one hand they were aware of "stranger danger" and sought known sperm donors whom they felt were less likely to be HIV positive. On the other hand, they often felt so grateful and indebted to the sperm donor that they did not always insist on HIV testing. One obvious conclusion that can be drawn from this study is that low-income women should have access to semen banking and fertility medicine services, so that they can use medically screened and quarantined sperm, and thereby reduce the risk of infection to themselves and their children. This could be considered a small-scale but important form of HIV prevention. All women, regardless of sexual orientation, should have access to sperm that is health-screened to reduce the rates of reproduction-related HIV transmission. Reproduction, after all, is not compatible with "safer sex."

I write this as a risk-averse person, especially when it comes to the possibility, however remote, of contracting a lethal infection. It bears noting, however, that the necessity of freezing and quarantining semen is far from proven. In fact, activists and scholars have offered devastating critiques of the standard semen quarantining practice (which is also the official recommendation of the ASRM). Nachtigall argues that using frozen and quarantined semen:

1. Approximately doubles the patient's cost of treatment
2. Reduces pregnancy rates by 50 percent
3. Reduces the number of pregnancies because of patient dropout
4. Leads to an ethically troubling increase in physician income as a direct result of the diminished efficacy of treatment
5. Has not been demonstrated to be necessary to prevent the transmission of HIV in AI.[16]

Other researchers note that only six documented cases of insemination-associated AIDS were reported to the CDCP between 1985 and 1996.[17] Many have noted that insemination is less likely than penile-vaginal intercourse to transmit the virus because the greater friction of the latter may cause micro-tears in vaginal tissues. Nachtigall concludes, "All available data suggest that neither safety nor efficacy need be sacrificed in the current practice of donor insemination by offering patients the choice of appropriately screened fresh or frozen sperm."[18] This argument is difficult for me to refute logically, although my gut feeling remains that quarantining the sperm is safer than not. Still, women considering or undergoing insemination have reason to seriously deliberate, given their age and financial constraints, whether fresh semen from an appropriately screened sperm donor might be their best option.

Putting into place basic legal protections for the family is also expensive. These legal processes are not only time consuming and frequently emotionally draining, but can cost in the thousands of dollars. The following documents are suggested by the National Center for Lesbian Rights (NCLR) and the Human Rights Campaign Fund's FamilyNet (HRCF) as necessary and basic for legal protection of lesbian families. Some help to protect the partnership of the parents, while others address the relationships among parents and children.

> Autopsy and Disposition of Remains
> Authorization for Consent to Medical Treatment of Minor
> Consent Forms for School, Travel, and Medical Decision-making
> Co-Parenting Agreement
> Directive to Physicians
> Domestic Partnership Agreement
> Donor Insemination Agreement
> Durable Power of Attorney for Finances
> Durable Power of Attorney for Health Care (and Addendum to
>   Durable Power of Attorney for Health Care)
> Health Care Proxy
> Hospital Visitation Authorization
> Last Will and Testament
> Living Will
> Nomination of Conservator of Estate/Person
> Nomination of Guardianship/Conservatorship for a Minor
> Revocation of Durable Power of Attorney
> Right to Receive Personal Property

These documents represent a maze of expensive, time-consuming, and second-class protections for lesbian families. All these rights are accorded automatically to married heterosexual parents and their children. Further, certain legal protections for families started with AI may hinge on the mediation of a physician in the insemination.

Lesbians with few financial resources are also discouraged from undertaking AI in less direct though equally prohibitive ways. One of the most important of these is that "doing" family costs money. In U.S. culture, family is associated with bourgeois activities and trappings. In an ethnographic study of fifty-two "lesbigay" households in the San Francisco Bay Area (evenly divided between male and female couples), sociologist Christopher Carrington found that those couples with more money were much more likely to consider themselves family, regardless of the longevity of their relationships.

> The ability to achieve familyhood is differentially distributed and the stark reality is that the affluent more easily, and more frequently, achieve that status for themselves.[19]

Carrington identifies domesticity as central to whether these LGBT couples see themselves as family, and whether others see them as family. Affluent families, he finds, are much more able to do (or pay someone else to do) the domestic work: cleaning, gardening, pet-care, "consumption work" such as shopping and vacationing, entertaining, cooking elaborate meals, gift-giving, celebrating holidays, visiting, and maintaining relationships with family. Doing these things makes same-sex couples feel like family.

> Clearly, domesticity becomes more comprehensive and ample among those with greater socioeconomic resources. Such families maintain more relationships, engage in more extensive social interaction and community participation, hold jobs offering more flexible time, possess more money to spend and consequently can invest more effort in the construction and maintenance of family. Those lesbigay families who possess these things lead richer, more fulfilling family lives.[20]

Since lesbian individuals and couples have lower incomes than (gay or straight) men, most lesbians lack the resources to create a family life rich in consumptive domesticity.

Lesbians of the liquid classes are much more likely to have the re-sources to "do" family in all its forms, including undertaking AI. Pursu-ing pregnancy can be seen as another family-building form of domestic-ity. It requires not only money but also time, energy, and sophisticated consumption and social skills.[21] Participating in the process of achieving pregnancy builds a sense of family not only if/when the inseminee be-comes pregnant, but in the multiple steps required to achieve pregnancy.

Carrington's study gives scant attention to the impact of children on "doing" family. Wealth and other forms of privilege endow families with cultural legitimacy less available to low-income lesbians, lesbians of color, and/or lesbians living with disabilities.[22] Nevertheless, lower-income lesbians can and do achieve pregnancy outside of the medical system. I would argue that having children, regardless of income, catapults lesbians into seeing themselves, their children, and their partners—and being seen by others—as family. Like other low-income families, they also shop, clean, cook, and maintain relationships. Whether through self-insemina-tion, by getting pregnant through PIVMO, or through informal adoption, lesbians find ways to "do" family with whatever resources they have.

Some of the barriers to insemination for low-income lesbians hinge on the vulnerability of all low-income women to the state when it comes to childbearing and childrearing. Low-income lesbians are not what legal scholar Ruthann Robson calls "but for" lesbians. "But for" lesbians are exactly like idealized heterosexuals but for the sex of their partners.[23] Be-cause low-income and poor lesbians are by definition not "but for" les-bians, they are far less likely to be deemed deserving of legal protections and services by courts, court-appointed social workers, physicians, and other officials. Because their exclusion from legal and cultural "legiti-macy" is basically pre-ordained, and because they have fewer financial re-sources to protect or fight over, low-income lesbians often do not invest their scarce resources in commodities such as frozen sperm, medically enhanced inseminations, and second-parent adoption.

Smaller, seemingly trivial inconveniences and disincentives also add up to make AI less attractive for low-income lesbians. If you use a fresh-sperm donor, you have to coordinate schedules to inseminate during your fer-tile window each month. This is especially challenging when you have a job with inflexible work hours, and/or have to rely on public transportation, as most low-income women do. Lesbians often have bad experiences with the health care system, which leads to a reluctance to deal with doctors.[24] Lesbians who are poor, of color, receiving welfare, immigrants, or otherwise stigmatized often compound these negative experiences exponentially.

Sperm is Cheap: Semen Banking

The practices of semen banking also attempt to organize and secure racial, cultural, sexual, familial, and other distinctions that fortify the phallic ego. Guarding against the dangerous proximity of flow (understood in the West as moral and social chaos),[25] semen is strictly controlled: inventoried, classified, ranked, and catalogued in a near-parody of ego-defensive efficiency. As medical sociologists Matthew Schmidt and Lisa Jean Moore (1998) point out, the practice of semen banking serves to institutionalize already existing masculinist hierarchies through the sorting, treating, and labeling of semen. Preferences for tall, Caucasian, muscular, college-educated, and heterosexual sperm donors are reinforced by semen banking practices.

One problem with sperm donor profiles is that the sperm donor may lie. People lie about themselves for a variety of reasons, conscious and unconscious. A sperm donor may be in denial about hereditary problems in his family's health history, or he may not know about them. Mental illness in particular is so stigmatized that many people never learn about the mentally ill in their family. Even if they do know, they may process that information in such a way as to find it irrelevant. A sperm donor may lie about his sexual history, because he does not want to think about it, or because he has convinced himself it does not matter. Finally, a sperm donor may realize that a certain aspect of his family medical history may disqualify him for sperm donation, and decide to lie because he wants the "job."

The discursive production of what I call "Übersemen" is mirrored by its material production through elaborate psycho-socio-physiological sperm donor screening as well as high-tech semen "treatments." In their 1998 study "Downloading a Dream Daddy," Schmidt and Moore coin the term "technosemen" to describe the multiple layers of mechanical and rhetorical intervention in sperm-banked semen:

> Semen analysis includes: sperm counts, morphology, motility testing, functional testing, and sperm washing ranging from the swim-up methods to Percoll or 2-step simple wash . . . Computer-assisted semen analysis (CASA)—which uses digital computer imaging devices connected to microscopes—is now available to conduct all of these tests.

Through these processes of technoscientific mediation, Schmidt and Moore argue that technosemen reinforces the stratification of men by race, education, and other markers of social class, in the service of sperm bank profitability. Semen banks "construct technosemen as less risky to consumers, as being able to create better children, taller, smarter, and more musical." Because this process intensifies and reifies these power differentials with rhetorical and visual technologies as well as biomedical ones, the term "übersemen" better captures the character of the final product.[26]

Not surprisingly, given the marketing strategies of sperm banks, gay male sperm donors are systematically excluded from most U.S. semen banks not oriented toward a LGBT clientele. This exclusion has been the official policy of the American Society for Reproductive Medicine since 1980.[27] Gay and bisexual men are viewed as members of a "high-risk group" and hence disallowed by most semen banks regardless of their individual HIV status or risk factors. That homosexual and bisexual men can be rejected as sperm donors because U.S. and European gay male communities have been among the hardest hit by the AIDS epidemic is convenient for semen banks, who can assure recipients that they use no (genetically tainted?) gay sperm donors.

While semen banking can be critiqued as commodified, alienated, dehumanizing and eugenic, in the context of lesbian baby-making, it is also in the process of being transformed into a more humane, or at least a significantly different, enterprise. Commercialization is chief among the issues that feminists and other ethicists have taken up in relation to procreative technologies. Many feminists, as well as conservative critics of contractual and technological procreation (e.g., Kimbrell 1993), have singled out the profit motive, and the assigning of a price to human life and procreation, as profound violations of the sanctity of human life. This criticism can certainly be applied to AI, particularly in its most institutionalized forms, in which semen is technologically manipulated as well as bought, sold, and profited from. Lesbian AI, however, may also be seen as part of a very different discourse from that of heteronormative, patriarchal, capitalist eugenics.

Charges of commodification in the process of AI, particularly lesbian AI, seem to me shortsighted. The term "commodification" is part of a Marxian discourse that implies a utopian prior and/or future time when exchange value, reification, the profit motive, and alienation were not/will not be present. Non-commodified exchange, on the other hand, elicits both socialist visions of use value, unalienated labor, production for need not profit, and organic visions of pre-capitalist gift exchange, potlatch, and a more generous sharing of boundaries.[28] Any of these may be vastly preferable to commodity capitalism, but none of them are realistic options for lesbians to wait for as they decide whether or not to have children. Lesbians (and other women) should also know to be wary of the romanticization of past "pre-commodified" economies. Women were and are not necessarily better off in kinship economies that do not parley in exchange and surplus values. That women, their procreative capacities, and their sexuality have long been the object of exchange in non-capitalist (as well as capitalist) economies is all too clear. As feminists have understood for many years, the notion that heterosexual babymaking is untainted by economics is naive.

Rather than simply locating alienated procreation in "commodification," one could argue that at least the commodification of procreation is accompanied by contracts, which, when women are a party to them, offer women a chance at agency. Ironically, when semen is commodified, that is, given an exchange value, women may gain increased procreative options. This gain is recognized in the gay and feminist celebrations of "choice," and in women's contradictory relationships to the market. The question is not so much a matter of whether economics will encroach on the body or the family, but rather what kinds of exchanges will take place, on what terms, for what purposes, and under whose control.

Many of the criticisms of the commercialization of women's procreative and sexual capacities do not apply to the commercialization of semen. First, there is no violation of bodily integrity in the collection of semen, unlike the "collection" of a woman's eggs, the use of her body in "surrogacy," or the commodification of her sexuality in most forms of prostitution. Rather, the production of a semen sample for sale or donation takes place in private, much like the production of a urine sample. Unlike donating human ova, "donating" sperm—at least as a physical process—is something the sperm donors would likely be doing anyway.[29] In fact, rather than requiring pay, many men will themselves pay for "better" masturbation, as they do for pornography and other masturbatory aids.

The class exploitation endemic to the commercialization of women's sexual and procreative capacities is also absent in the current social relations of AI. Whereas most women who trade sex for money, drugs, meals, or a place to stay are extremely economically marginalized and socially vulnerable, eugenic discourses that underlie AI ironically ensure that the semen "worth paying for" on the open market is the semen of the socioeconomic elite.[30] The semen most preferred by buyers is that of men who are white, healthy, and college educated. Semen produced by men who are too poor to have gone to college, who have health problems due to poverty, or who are disproportionately affected by HIV infection, drug use, hepatitis, TB, and many other "poor people's illnesses" are automatically excluded from semen donation.

I see little problem continuing to pay men for their semen if they are willing to sell it, even for those who hold an ethical position that rejects the sale of body parts or the commercialization of human eggs or the rental of wombs. Attaching the element of contract to the semen exchange strengthens the argument that the sperm donor is not a father, and therefore should not be given paternal status or rights.[31] This protection is important to many inseminating lesbians, including many who want to keep open the possibility that their child(ren) might eventually know their sperm donor. The sale of women's procreative capacities is often injurious and exploitative. The demographics of semen sperm donors ensure that sperm selling has little danger of exploiting impoverished or otherwise vulnerable men.

Putting semen into the cold calculus of supply-side economics makes it overwhelmingly evident that semen is not a priceless commodity, but is in fact the most readily renewable bodily product on the market. In fact, a man can sell his semen more frequently than he can sell his blood. Commercializing semen means recognizing how available and "cheap" it is (at current rates, one can buy approximately ten to fifteen thousand sperm for a penny).[32] Choosing to "donate" (sell) one's sperm to strangers is simply another option for generating income that one is free to pursue. The shifts in patrilineal norms among the liquid classes,[33] and of men's historic concern with passing on name and property to offspring, are so complete that men freely "cast their seed to the wind," perhaps siring broods of children who will all be strangers, with full legal and medical sanction.[34] Men have always cast about their seed beyond the marital circle. Engels noted this fact when he wrote that female prostitution has always been the semi-acknowledged companion of "civilized" marriage.[35]

The reasons men give for reluctance or refusal to sell their sperm often pertain to a less atomized and more socially "connected" discourse of kinship. They do not want to have children in the world about whose existence they do not know, and with whom they have no relationship.[36] Yet the phenomenon of male participation in AI, while numerically small, is culturally and socially significant. It reflects both the ultra-commodification of all aspects of life in the postmodern moment, and the cultural acceptability of men's alienation from their offspring.

The sale of sperm also indicates growing biotechnologization of our understanding of our bodies. The man who sells his semen for forty dollars a specimen is not attributing to his sperm many of the meanings feudal men presumably did (e.g., as transmitting his place in a naturalistic social order). Rather, he sees a biological potentiality, with an exchange value, in whose future he is not invested. His market-alienation from his offspring has reached a level that few of his forefathers could have imagined. He has fully separated the social (being a "dad") from the biological (providing sperm) and the sexual (having PIVMO with a fertile woman). This separation, and its social sanction, takes place in a historical context in which biology has both lost and gained its power to define kinship. Lesbian AI could only have emerged out of the context these developments provide.

The separation of social reproduction from biological reproduction has long been men's prerogative. Under the law, men have historically enjoyed the option of legally recognizing extramarital offspring, and fatherhood remains primarily a legal status while motherhood almost always flows from biology.[37] This alienation of fatherhood is hardly unique to our historical moment. What is new is men's ability to become non-legal, yet biological, fathers for cash rather than for sexual reasons. This continuing male separation of the biological from the social occurs as the male flight from families with children continues to accelerate and as adult manhood is defined increasingly by norms of radical individualism, "freedom" from kinship or other interpersonal loyalties, signs of sexual prowess, and capital accumulation and consumption.[38] Yet a defining difference between AI and all other forms of assisted and contractual procreation is that with AI, it is men, not women, who are commodifying their body parts, and disaggregating (alienating) their procreative capacities from their sexual operations.

Internationally, a score of studies on the attitudes of sperm donors has been published. They are primarily survey-based and focus on what percentages would like their identity to be known to their offspring, whether they would "donate" if they weren't paid, and similar important but limited questions.[39] As one might expect, sperm donors have a range of motivations for providing sperm. Social scientist Ken Daniels summarizes the findings of the twenty-three studies of sperm donor attitudes from France, the United Kingdom, the United States, Canada, Australia, New Zealand, Denmark, Belgium, and Czechoslovakia.

> Altruistic reasons or financial reward, or some combination of the two, is what most semen providers report as being their reasons for becoming involved. Three other reasons appear in some of the studies: the desire to test one's own fertility; a desire to procreate; and sexual satisfaction.[40]

In teasing apart the motivations of sperm donors, "age, marital status, children, occupation, and reasons for providing semen are interlinked."[41] Altruistic motivations are associated with sperm donors who are older, married or in stable relationships, have children of their own, and are in professional occupations. Financial motivations, not surprisingly, are associated with sperm donors who are younger, unattached to a stable relationship, have no children of their own, and are students. Different kinds of recruiting practices seem to attract sperm donors with differing motivations: The social construction of semen donation as a commercial practice attracts sperm donors in sync with that view, and discourages others.[42]

Sperm donors are far more open to being contacted by future offspring than is generally believed by physicians. Many sperm donors would like, at a minimum, to know whether any children resulted from inseminations using their sperm. As Daniels summarizes:

> [I]t is clear that the majority of semen providers in many different countries in the world, and operating within different clinic policies, wish to have information concerning the outcomes of their contributions.[43]

Perhaps in part because in the vast majority of cases no such knowledge or contact is allowed, a number of authors are finding that some sperm donors have regrets about having participated.[44] There has not yet been any study of known sperm donors, or of known sperm donors to lesbian families in particular. These limitations make it difficult to generalize findings to the situation of lesbian AI except in broad strokes.

Lesbian-centered AI is Anti-patriarchal

The commercialization of semen, far from being an exploitative social practice, serves to demystify semen and (ejaculatory) fatherhood in ways that can be seen as feminist and socially progressive. While the commodification of semen can be contained readily within a modernist discourse of differentiation and disenchantment, its use by lesbians, I believe, cannot. Once again, we see lesbians (and their collaborators) shuffling the (stacked) semiotic deck, dealing a different kind of hand.

By taking a woman-centered rather than a married-couple-centered approach, the discourses and practices of self-insemination challenge the whole conglomeration of ideologies and power relations that characterize the patriarchal family. Alternative insemination is no longer about "treating" or compensating for the infertility of the husband in a married couple. Rather, AI is the provision of a product (viable sperm) to a woman who has made a decision to become pregnant. The technology of AI becomes an anti-patriarchal force.

Alternative insemination, as such, materially separates sexuality from procreation. Like contraception, it puts an element of choice into the procreative process that otherwise allegedly would be under the exclusive control of God or Nature.[45] It bestows on individuals (women) choices that in former times were simply unavailable in the same way.[46] Nowhere in this picture is the phallic notion of pregnancy in which women are seen as receptacles for men's "seed." Rather the patriarchal concept of the father is seriously problematized. And, perhaps most extraordinary, women, not heterosexual couples or men, become the standard in their procreative decision-making.

In the essay translated as "Commodities among Themselves," French philosopher Luce Irigaray offers a model for lesbian economy, which supplies a useful analytic tool for conceptualizing lesbian AI. Irigaray theorizes what she calls "subversive commerce," a female economics not containable within the symbolics of either (phallic) capitalism or (phallic) "gift exchange." Irigaray uses the work of Claude Lévi-Strauss ("father" of anthropology) and Sigmund Freud ("father" of psychology) in order to pursue the feminist theories she finds inherent, yet suppressed, in their "findings." With Jacques Lacan, her rejected former teacher, she appropriates from Lévi-Strauss both the exchange of women in the "gift economy" of "primitive" kinship relations and Lévi-Strauss' misogynist and unimaginative assertion that neither culture nor language could exist without the exchange of women among men.[47] She takes to task Freud's inability to deal with either his lesbian patients or the subject of lesbian existence without resorting to reductive (phallic) homologies that render lesbians invisible/impossible, as merely "masculine" or possessed of "male libidinal energies." Irigaray remarks on Freud and Lévi-Strauss' negation of even the possibility of female agency, particularly in its lesbian forms.

> Female homosexuality . . . is recognized only to the extent that it is *prostituted to man's fantasies.* Commodities can only enter into relationships under the watchful eyes of their "guardians." It is out of the question for them to go to "market" on their own, enjoy their own worth among themselves, speak to each other, and desire each other, free from the control of seller-buyer-consumer subjects. And the interests of businessmen require that commodities relate to each other as rivals.[48]

This passage suggests the possibility of lesbians subverting the business-as-usual of men's (commercial) fantasies of women as objects.

This formulation is remarkably aligned with that put forth in the U.S. feminist classic "The Traffic in Women: Notes on the 'Political Economy' of Sex" by anthropologist Gayle Rubin. Seeking to illuminate the "relationships whereby a female becomes a woman," Rubin's essay also used Freud and Lévi-Strauss via Lacan to formulate a psycho-socio-economic model for understanding the subordination of women.[49] What she emerged with was the "sex/gender system." The sex/gender system was, of course, the theory that separated the physiological (sex) from the culturally imposed meanings of that biological difference (gender), and thus formed a cornerstone of feminist theorizing and politics ever since. Because this formulation was so revolutionary, and has been used widely by feminist theorists (and many others) since its publication, Rubin's thinking bears quoting at length:

> The needs of sexuality and procreation must be satisfied as much as the need to eat, and . . . these needs are hardly ever satisfied in any "natural" form, any more than are the needs for food. Hunger is hunger, but what counts as food is culturally determined and obtained. . . . Sex is sex, but what counts as sex is equally culturally determined and obtained. Every society also has a sex/gender system—a set of arrangements by which the biological raw material of human sex and procreation is shaped by human, social intervention and satisfied in a conventional manner, no matter how bizarre some of the conventions may be.[50]

In Rubin's formulation, "sex" is the biological fact of femaleness or maleness, and "gender" is the norms of femininity and masculinity that a given society teaches are based "naturally" on sex. Rubin's articulation of the sex/gender system has been used productively by feminists for more than a quarter of a century, and has become subject to feminist revisions over the years. The explanatory power and analytical importance of this seemingly simple distinction is still thrown into sharp relief by the seeming inability of many people, including the medical profession, to differentiate between the two terms. An article in the prestigious *Journal of Fertility and Sterility* discusses the ethics of (the misnomer) "preconception gender selection" rather than the (accurate) term "preconception sex selection."[51]

The continuing importance of the sex/gender distinction is also evident in the ongoing battles over "gender rights" and "sexual rights" at the international level. In attempts to prevent women's human rights from being enshrined in official UN documents, fundamentalist religious groups have labored to cast "gender" as a code word for lesbianism, and thus used lesbian-baiting to turn popular opinion against "gender equality" and "gender rights."[52] Opponents of women's human rights have also endeavored to control the definition of "gender" so that it can only refer to "men and women" and therefore not encompass women's rights to bodily, reproductive, and sexual integrity that would normally inhere to "gender rights."

En route to the sex/gender system, Rubin articulated what is one of the most intelligible English language interpretations of some of the feminist implications of "the phallus" in Lacanian psychoanalysis. While I would not presume to summarize these implications, a few excerpts go a long way toward illuminating a subject perceived as esoteric by many U.S. academics.

> Lacan makes a . . . radical distinction between the penis and the "phallus," between organ and information . . . The presence or absence of the phallus carries the differences between two sexual statuses, "man" and "woman" . . . The phallus also carries the meaning of the difference between "exchanger" and "exchanged," gift and giver. . . . In the cycle of exchange manifested by the oedipal complex, the phallus passes through the medium of women from one man to another . . . Women go one way, the phallus the other. *It is where we aren't.* In this sense, the phallus is more than a feature that distinguishes the sexes; it is the embodiment of the male status, to which men accede and in which certain rights inhere—among them, the right to a woman. [Emphasis Rubin's.][53]

Like Rubin, Irigaray focuses in on the incipient theory of sexual subjection in the (evidently misogynist) works of Freud and Lévi-Strauss. Perhaps more importantly, she locates and elaborates its more or less equally obscured twin theory of sexual de-subjection, or "liberation." Against the texts of Lévi-Strauss and Freud, Irigaray asserts lesbian subjectivity as representing a crisis in phallic symbolic economies. If women are commodity-objects to be exchanged among men, how then to explain agential lesbian existence? And what if these "commodities" refused to go to "market"? What if they maintained "another" kind of commerce, among themselves? Irigaray responds to these (her own) questions with a utopian discourse of lesbian exchanges that are not outside of, but rather are rupturing of, dominant symbolics.

> Exchanges without identifiable terms, without accounts, without end . . . Without additions and accumulations, one plus one, woman after woman . . . Without sequence of number. Without standard or yardstick . . . As for all the strategies and savings, the appropriations tantamount to theft and rape, the laborious accumulation of capital, how ironic all that would be.[54]

Irigaray conceives of lesbianism itself as a form of "subversive commerce" that potent(ial)ly undermines patriarchy.

Along similar lines, lesbian AI can also be seen as a form of subversive commerce: not outside of, but radically disruptive of, the phallic symbolic economy in which it takes place. On the Oedipal front, lesbian AI disrupts the phallic narrative and its psychic brutality, which ostensibly shapes us into little boys and girls. For instance, lesbian motherhood spares daughters the devaluing of the female (e.g., "castration trauma"), which Freud and his descendents would have us believe leads her to disparage her mother and her own sex in favor of men. Perhaps even more dramatically, having one or two lesbian mothers interrupts the Freudian narrative that teaches that a girl is "castrated" in relation to her father, that she can never "have" a woman "of her own," and that maleness is somehow more desirable than femaleness.

In contrast to Freudian and Lévi-Straussian narratives, the lesbian AI mother can both "have" and "give away" the phallus. That is, she has the power to exchange (as opposed to being the currency of exchange) in kinship. She "has" a woman "of her own" and in fact could be said to reverse the flow of phallic power. Power ceases to flow in circuits Irigaray calls "hom(m)o-sexual" (e.g., from man to man, through the bodies of women).[55] Instead, the inseminating lesbian exchanges power (semen) on terms to which she is party. Her relation to men does not define her (lesbian) kinship status. Nor is her mothering part of a discourse of the circulation of women, children, objects, and signs among men.

The lesbian AI mother thus claims "phallic" prerogatives in profoundly threatening ways. Most obviously she claims them sexually. She almost certainly claims them economically, in the financial self-sufficiency generally required of lesbians (and increasingly of all women).[56] And she claims them always in terms of kinship, where she, as Irigaray might say, has gone to market. She has broken with the (phallic) propriety of both proper names and property. She will pass on her own name to her children, or a name she negotiates with her lesbian partner, her children's other mother. She has become proprietary, purchasing semen, "having a woman." She is thoroughly "inappropriate."

The inseminating lesbian, however, is not exterior to, and has not made a break from, the patriarchy. Her "own" name, of course, comes from her father, unless she (or her mother) has changed it, and the concept of a proper name itself is thoroughly patriarchal, another mechanism to lubricate the passage of property down the legally legitimated paternal "line." The lesbian AI mother, like most of us, is both proprietary and property, variously located in the grids of class exploitation. Finally, she is both appropriate and inappropriate, accumulating a range of statuses through various identities and acts. In fact, some have argued that the positive status attributed to motherhood, as a fulfillment of femininity, cancels out or even overrides the negative status of lesbianism.[57] As with each of these oppositions, it is rarely so simple, since neither lesbian nor mother is a completed identity. Each is significantly transformed by co-axes of class, race, ethnicity, (dis)ability, and a host of other marked identity classifications in particular national and cultural contexts.

Lesbian AI can be seen as a form of positive, subversive commerce, even within the wide range of positions that feminists have taken regarding Lacan's theory of the phallus.[58] Despite lesbian AI's less-than-total break from phallic signifying systems, or perhaps because of its oppositional and radical interiority to them, it disrupts them on symbolic, cultural, and institutional fronts.

6

Transforming the Means of Reproduction
Lesbian AI Kinship and Politics

ABSTRACT

In this chapter, I discuss how lesbian AI transforms lesbian kinship and politics, which in turn transform each other. I discuss how lesbians have negotiated the complex social and medical terrain of the infertility industry, transforming it and being transformed by it in turn.

Lesbian-Feminism

Lesbians have always been central to feminism, in all known feminist movements. Lesbian-feminism, however, is a particular politics that understands lesbianism as an act of resistance to patriarchy, and as a prefiguration of a feminist future. Conversely, kinship practices in intentional lesbian families have profoundly affected lesbian-feminist politics.

Early in the lesbian baby boom alternative insemination was understood as part of a lesbian-feminist politics that challenged male domination and promoted progressive social change. As philosopher Anne Ferguson wrote,

> We . . . require autonomous women's networks that maintain women's independent leadership of the fight against male dominance. We also need to choose lifestyles which symbolize the independence of women from male service such as feminist communal living, co-habitation rather than marriage, gay/lesbian/bisexual lifestyles, artificial insemination and adoption, single parenting, and so forth.[1]

Lesbian-feminism enjoyed an explosion of popularity in the 1970s, although it fell from grace in the so called "lesbian sex wars" of the 1980s. Lesbian-feminism sees lesbian existence as a political position at the vanguard of the radical feminist movement.

In this context, AI was understood as a form of lesbian empowerment, enabling lesbians to conceive, bear, and rear children without fathers. It was a practice inflected by lesbian separatism, with a significant part of the appeal being that one virtually did not have to deal with any men whatsoever. If one used a female go-between to procure the semen, even contact with a male donor was unnecessary.

Lesbian separatism was an important part of the lesbian-feminist movement. While understandings and practices differed, separatism was based on the belief that men and their institutions had a parasitic relationship to women. In a patriarchal society, women could not be liberated in the company of men. Instead, by separating themselves from men, they could pour their untapped gynergy into other women, thus engendering a feminist counterculture that prioritized women's concerns and women's liberation.

To this end, lesbian-feminists created a multiplicity of "women's spaces" to live, be, love, smash the patriarchy, and create feminist realities free from the encumbering presence of men. In its heyday in the United States, these spaces included women's coffeehouses, rape crisis centers, music festivals, poetry readings, self-defense collectives, study groups, printing presses, newspapers and newsletters, communal households, health clinics, women's studies courses and programs, restaurants, music labels, consciousness-raising groups, bookstores, childcare collectives, take-back-the-night marches, covens, and "womyn's land" to name a few. And yes, alternative insemination, procreation, and parenting without men were celebrated as well.

Each of these physical and cultural spaces created related psychic spaces for lesbian women. This was a time of incredible productivity for feminist thought and activism. For many, it was possible to live a woman-centered life in a way that was simply unimaginable a few years earlier. Despite their utopianism, or perhaps because of it, many of these women's spaces contained the seeds of their own destruction. It was not long before the euphoria of political symbiosis gave way to the disappointments and battles of lesbian differences. Lesbians fought about all kinds of things: politics, race, class, sadomasochism, pornography, political strategy, feminism, and separatism.

As the fortunes of lesbian-feminism shifted, so did lesbian AI. Where lesbian political culture in the 1970s was more separatist, in the 1980s we shifted toward close involvement with lesbians' "gay brothers." Impelled in large part by the HIV/AIDS crisis, lesbians began to make common cause with gay men to fight for resources, education, and care for gay men sick with HIV disease. Where a few years earlier, lesbian discourse had emphasized gender-separatism, now we saw the growth of LGBT and "queer" consciousness, with the political movement relevant to lesbians also including gay men.

"Queer" consciousness and activism grew out of the post-Stonewall, post-gay-liberation, post-lesbian-feminist 1980s. It represented both an unprecedented level of coalition between lesbians and gay men and an unprecedented level of cynicism and retrenchment spurred by the Reagan era. This was played out against the backdrop of AIDS, the backlash against feminism, the so-called lesbian sex wars, and the attacks on "political correctness" in the larger social context of massive militarization, social spending cuts, and government corruption, all proliferating in a climate of political deception. Queer politics expressed the utter rage and frustration of gay men and lesbians around murderous government indifference to the AIDS crisis.

Queer politics marks one side of a long term split in LGBT political activity and in the ways LGBT people conceptualize their communities that goes back at least to the nineteenth century, when the term "homosexual" first emerged. The opposition between homophile and transgressive social movements characterizes this split. Where homophilism can be characterized by the desire to assimilate, transgressive movements can be seen as forms of nationalist separatism.

The homophile position holds the view that homosexuals are just like anybody else, except that they happen to be attracted to people of the same sex. Oppression of LGBT people is seen as an irrational form of discrimination against people who just happen to love differently. Along with this position go attempts to convince the straight world that they have nothing to fear from us because we are more similar to them then we are different. Homophile politics constitutes a plea for acceptance.

Queer politics, on the other hand, is the militant assertion of difference. Queer politics acknowledges the role of gender as a means of social control and attempts to radically subvert it. Its in-your-face dramatics are offensive to many and thrilling to some. Rejecting the homophile position that we are "just like" straight people, queer politics asserts that we *are* different, are queer, are a threat to the order of things, and it demands respect for these differences.

As hated and reviled as gender transgressions are by much of the straight world, lesbians (and gay men) often internalize feelings of shame and self-hatred specifically around those aspects of their lives and communities that play with gender crossing, at the same time that they celebrate them.

Poet and scholar Judy Grahn points out how LGBT people have played a crucial role in many cultures across the globe and throughout history, often crossing proscribed gender boundaries into dangerous worlds of power and pleasure. Some scholars argue that such "queer" gender transgressions have roots in sacred traditions around the world that date back to ancient times.[2] The queer movement proudly reclaims this legacy of difference, and celebrates our unique gifts and perspectives as outsiders, at the same time that it gives agency to the rage engendered by centuries of oppression and violence. Unfortunately, queer politics, like nationalist movements in general, tend to privilege a single, in this case "queer," identity over all others, thus rigidifying qualifications for inclusion while marginalizing the concerns of those who have more complex identifications, such as women and people of color.

The shift in alliances from lesbian-feminism to queer politics was not universal, nor was it linear. In fact, the distinctions between the two movements and identities can be blurry. Many lesbians continued to be aligned politically and affectively with the women's movements, and eschewed connections with gay men. Many lesbians strongly felt that the AIDS crisis was yet another case of men (this time gay men) vampirizing women's (this time lesbian women's) precious energy. Other lesbians never stopped being identified with mixed-sex gay and lesbian communities. In working-class communities and communities of color in particular, bars and other meeting places had remained mixed-sex throughout the 1970s, and continued so through the 1980s and beyond.

Still, a sea change occurred in the practices of AI among lesbians. One effect was that lesbians became much more likely to want to use gay men as sperm donors. This change was affected sharply by the emergence of the HIV epidemic in male gay and bisexual communities. After 1982, lesbians' use of gay male sperm donors dropped off precipitously.[3]

The epidemic also contributed to the medicalization of AI among lesbians, as fear of contracting HIV inclined more lesbians to opt for screened sperm from sperm banks. In a less direct, but still powerful way, the AIDS crisis intensified the feeling among many lesbians of wanting to have children themselves, as if the creation of new life somehow made more bearable the ravages of AIDS in LGBT communities. Author and Chicana lesbian activist Cherríe Moraga writes of learning, within twenty-four hours, that a close friend is ill with AIDS and that the fetus she is carrying is a boy.

> Ella calls from work and tells me Tede is sick with AIDS. It is news I
> have been resisting for three days. A rumor, I told myself. But today it is
> confirmed, and I think only of the other news, of the boy I am to birth.
> There is meaning in the fact that my fetus has formed itself into a male,
> a meaning I must excavate from the most buried places in myself, as well
> as from this city [San Francisco], this era of dying into which my baby
> will be born.[4]

While Moraga was already pregnant when she learned of her friend's illness, the connection between the two facts is meaningful to her, as it is to many who experience themselves as carrying life in the midst of death.

Known Sperm Donors

Another way that AI changed in the 1980s is that lesbians became more concerned with the importance of fathers to their children or potential children. In the early years of lesbian AI, those considering it assumed that, because men weren't important in their lives, they wouldn't be important to their children either. After a number of years of seeing children grow up in the lesbian community, it became apparent that many children cared a lot about the paternal side of their origins.[5] This dawning awareness led those considering AI to think differently about the sperm donor role and how they wanted to negotiate it.

Debates raged internationally, both within and outside of the lesbian community, about contractual and technological procreation. Questions arose about the social and psychological ramifications of sperm donor anonymity, with some asserting that the ability to know one's genetic origins is a human right.[6] Mothers-to-be moved greatly in the direction of wanting known sperm donors for their children both in Europe and the United States and often wanting them to play a role in their children's and their own lives.[7]

Medical sociologist Laura Mamo conducted in-depth interviews with thirty-six lesbians from the San Francisco Bay Area, which she supplemented with observations of support groups for lesbians seeking to become parents. She also interviewed several service providers who work with lesbians seeking pregnancy. Mamo asked, "What are the most important qualities women in the Bay Area consider when choosing a donor from a sperm bank?" She found that:

> The elements considered most include first, a donor who is "willing to be known" to the offspring; second, a donor who has a "good" health status; third, a donor from a desired "racial/ethnic background"; and, fourth, a donor who shares social and cultural affinities with the potential parents.[8]

Valuing a known sperm donor opened up another realm of complexities in negotiating family relationships. As before, the sperm donor role was and is understood as a role open to negotiation.

Since the late 1960s, lesbians have created a vibrant if beleaguered institutional infrastructure that supports their dignity, their communities, their rights, and their survival. In response to the unsatisfactory situation in the mainstream medical establishment and in conventional sperm-banking practices, lesbians have created and sustained a number of lesbian-oriented procreative services, including sperm banks.

Several semen banks currently exist that are geared specifically toward lesbians, as well as sometimes toward single women, gay men, and other "alternative families." While these institutions necessarily share common ground with more conventional fertility service providers, they also offer services that stem from a uniquely lesbian perspective.

This perspective is reflected in the offerings of lesbian-oriented, feminist, and gay-friendly sperm banks, which provide some level of "known donor" options. The feminist and gay infertility services that¹ ʳe their own sperm banks—including the Sperm Bank of California (TSBC), Pacific Reproductive Services (PRS), and Rainbow Flag Health Services— all offer "known donor" options to recipients. These range from TSBC's offering of "yes" sperm donors, who agree to be known to their offspring when they reach the age of eighteen, to Rainbow Flag's stipulation that sperm donors and inseminating women be willing to be known to each other when the child reaches three months of age.[9]

All of the above provide the option of bringing your own sperm donor, but when they provide the donor the spectrum is wide. In addition to anonymous sperm donors, TSBC has what they call "identity release donors," whose identifying information will be given to the child at age eighteen on the child's request. Their motto: "We're a full-service semen bank."

Pacific Reproductive Services has a higher disclosure expectation for their known donors: They suggest a one-time meeting between child and sperm donor after the child reaches adulthood, again at the child's request only. Rainbow Flag has no anonymous donors at all. The bank always tells the mother who the sperm donor is when the child is three months old, and asks her to contact him by the time the child is a year old.[10] Although TSBC's website prominently features its practice of identity release, only a minority of its sperm donors are willing to participate in the practice. Of the twenty-one sperm donors currently listed as available on the Sperm Bank of California website, eight (38%) are "yes donors" and 13 (62%) are "no donors."[11]

One of the great distinctions between these providers and the rest of the AI universe is that lesbian-oriented services are concerned about the sperm donor's relationship with the child. This concern for the psychological well-being of children who may have an unknown biological parent is long standing among lesbians, and has been growing over time.[12] This concern is well articulated, particularly by lesbians who were themselves adopted, or who relinquished children for adoption. The National Lesbian Family Study (NLFS), a longitudinal study of lesbians who started their families with AI, found that "although three-quarters of the children in the study had no fathers, most mothers expected the children to grow up in the company of good, loving men. After their children were born, some mothers regretted having used unknown donors, and felt sad about the lost opportunity for their children to know their donor fathers."[13] Concerns about the potentially life-long impact on a child's psyche of not knowing her biological father seem to be common in the lesbian community.[14]

Research that might substantiate, or disprove, these concerns has been hard to come by, as studies of AI offspring are scant and often have been methodologically compromised. Most studies do not differentiate between children who are deceived about their conception and/or biological father, children raised with full knowledge of their origins, and children who learn of their origins later in life. This problem parallels the flaws of early studies of children's reactions to their parents' homosexuality, which failed to differentiate those raised by two stable same-sex parents from those whose mother (or father) came out later in life, often divorcing the other parent in the process.

Emerging evidence about lesbian AI indicates that the children born from this procedure are quite well adjusted, as one might expect in a family arrangement with much-wanted children and organized parents. Still, concerns about the children's psychological well-being often lead lesbians to want a known donor/father for their child.[15]

We know from the experience of adopted children in the United States that the psychosocial and identity issues they face may be profound and long-standing.[16] Some children with anonymous sperm donors may experience similar issues. The limited data about AI offspring is all based on children with anonymous sperm donors, and so should not be generalized to those who have a known father/sperm donor. Research on AI children of heterosexuals suggest that they may have feelings of loss due to not knowing their sperm donor, anger at him for abandoning them and for the conditions of their conception, anger at their mother, and painful difficulties around identity and belonging.[17] Again, this is in heterosexual-parent families, where the dynamics are quite different than in lesbian-parent families.

A Belgian study of forty-one children born to lesbian-parent AI families with unknown sperm donors reveals a small majority (56%) of children (who were between the ages of seven and seventeen) preferring no additional contact or information about the sperm donor. The rest of the children wanted to know more about their sperm donor. Most of these (27%) wanted to know his identity, and the remaining (19%) wanted specific kinds of non-identifying information. Several were interested in his appearance and whether they looked like him, while some wanted to know about his personality. Two children were interested in the process of the donation, and certain desires were mentioned only once: the sperm donor's age, birthday, hobbies, occupation, and whether he was still alive. Boys were much more likely than girls to want to meet their sperm donor. The children were twice as likely as their mothers to want information about the sperm donor.[18]

Some of these children accept and feel gratitude toward the sperm donor. They may experience mild to intense curiosity about him, accept his lack of role in their lives, or even feel indifferent.[19]

Barbara Raboy, former director of TSBC, was interviewed for an ABC News 20/20 segment on the topic of AI and its emotional effects on offspring (19, January 1998). Raboy noted that awareness about the impact on the children of anonymous sperm donors is growing.

> I think for a long time people were thinking, All I care about is getting pregnant. And the sperm banks were thinking, All we care about is getting the product out so that she can get pregnant. Now people are thinking more, I'm going to have a kid out there. A live human being with feelings and probably questions. What do I owe that child? Whereas 20 years ago, it was, I won't tell my child anything.[20]

TSBC is one of the leaders in offering the option of a known sperm donor. As of the late 1990s, 40 percent of their sperm donors were "yes donors," and 80 percent of their clients wished to use a "yes donor."[21] Other organizations facilitating known-donor lesbian AI include the Prospective Queer Parents (PQP) website, which "posts ads for people

seeking parenting or known–donor arrangements with other queer prospective parents," and the Conception Connection, "a network of lesbians and gay men who are looking for partners of the opposite sex with
whom to have biological children."

Prospective Queer Parents is an organization with a do-it-yourself at-
titude toward finding potential partners in creating children. PQP has
a web page on which it posts advertisements of "queer" people of any
gender who wish to be in some kind of co-parenting arrangement with
someone of the other sex. The idea is that both parties will not only
know their offspring, but will actively participate in parenting in a way
that meets both of their needs. The ads are not screened, simply sorted
for geographical area, including "Willing to relocate/Geographically
flexible," Australia, Canada, the Netherlands, the U.K., and thirty U.S.
states. In this forum, lesbians seek a spectrum of men from "donor" to
"dad." These ads can get pretty creative. The web page includes inquiries
from prospective parents in a variety of situations:

> A single lesbian looking for an uninvolved Euro-American donor;
> A lesbian couple looking for a First Nations (Native American)
> donor;
> A gay male couple looking for limited involvement with a "pro-
> fessional" lesbian co-mother;
> A single gay man looking for a local woman, or women, with
> whom to co-parent.[22]

The ads articulate interests in a wide range of family arrangements,
from sperm donation to cooperative parenting, from occasional contact
to living together, in the country, the city, and the suburbs. Reading these
ads, I am impressed by the sincerity, uniqueness, and complexity of each
individual and couple who seeks to parent, and the extent to which they
have articulated their parenting needs and desires. This diversity in desired parenting arrangements is a hallmark of ultramodernity, with the
hegemonic family system giving way to a plethora of individualized family formations, with the role of the donor (but not the mother) understood as open to negotiation. These prospective parents have clearly done
a great deal of soul-searching. They also seem exceptionally clear about
what compromises they are willing, and unwilling, to make.

If PQP is the personal ads of lesbian and gay parenting, the Conception Connection is the dating service. The Conception Connection works quite differently from PQP because it is mediated. The Conception Connection serves lesbian and gay clients who wish to be biological parents. Again, the expectations run the gamut from barely-known donor to full co-parent. It is directed by a lesbian social worker, who does an intake, including a detailed questionnaire, for each potential parent, and then exchanges anonymous profiles of those in the connection that might be a match. If it looks like a potential match to both parties, she then shares full names and phone numbers. If they still feel ready to go ahead, the director does extensive counseling to make sure their expectations really match, and medical, legal, and logistical issues are all well addressed. Because of the extensive services, many find the Conception Connection to be much safer than personal ads. It does, of course, cost money — currently $3,000.[23]

The spectrum between having a "yes donor" who will be known to your child when she turns eighteen and an actively parental father is wide. But all these alternatives stand in stark contrast to the overwhelming majority of non-lesbian inseminations, which are performed with the sperm of an anonymous donor, and with children not told of their origins. This emphasis on known sperm donors reflects and shapes lesbian baby-making practices.

Whether using a semen bank, or choosing a friend to co-parent, lesbians may use physical appearance in their donor selections to reinforce kinship. It would be reductive to perceive this as simply eugenics among lesbians, although that also may be involved. Rather, as Kath Weston argues,

> Heterosexual couples, too, often sought their union and reflection in their children, with comments about which parent a child "takes after" in looks, likes, or behavior. Yet the situation of lesbian mothers choosing a donor for insemination differed in that they could very deliberately select for certain physical characteristics, sometimes in a conscious attempt to reinforce the legally vulnerable tie to a lover.[24]

By drawing on the social significance that infuses notions of biology, a lesbian couple can effectively make a statement about who constitutes the child's "real" parents.

In lesbian AI, trying to control the appearance of one's children may speak of eugenic social control, but also, paradoxically, of lesbian empowerment. Lesbians, in this case, are appropriating "the natural" from its metaphysical "home" in patriarchal discourse. Lesbian appropriation of the natural-maternal is not necessarily a nostalgic gesture or a straight-forward conservative move. It is yet another way that lesbian baby-making shuffles the discursive deck so long stacked against lesbians, replacing signifiers of denigration with valorized ones that support lesbian autonomy and AI families. In such a prototypically "postmodern" shuffling of signifiers, things are no longer what they seem. In the midst of the lesbian baby boom, we can't know, looking at a pregnant woman, whether her maternity means adherence to heteronormative conventions or its opposite, a third term that is neither of the above, or a pastiche of all of them. The lesbian mother, continuing the semiotic disruption occasioned by the "single mother," has destabilized the referent at the basis of sexual difference (the feminine mother), thus putting up for grabs all the chains of meaning that were formerly linked to it.

By expanding access to women who are normally excluded from the AI practices of infertility specialists, self-insemination and pro-lesbian sperm banks democratize access to sperm outside of marriage, although cost is still a prohibitive factor for many women.

Some lesbian-oriented AI providers are also sensitive to the eugenic implications of semen banking, and aim for less eugenic criteria in their donor descriptions. At least one provider explicitly welcomes gay donors, who are typically eschewed by semen banks as a "high risk group."[25] Some provide a more racially and ethnically diverse donor list, and some offer semen from men who admit to small physiological or psychological problems such as a deviated septum or mild Attention Deficit Disorder.[26] Some provide more qualitative descriptions of the donors—with the probably unintended effect of making them seem like personal ads for a mate with descriptors such as "dreamer" and "soulful eyes." Some emphasize support services for recipients, careful donor-recipient matchmaking, instruction in self-insemination, and home delivery of frozen semen. Rainbow Flag Health Services has a unique approach. Along with offering exclusively gay, known donors, they take a strong stand against what they consider to be child abuse, and refuse to inseminate anyone who plans to circumcise their children or use corporal punishment.

More can be known about sperm donors, so more is known. Lesbians perusing sperm bank catalogues and menus of sperm-manipulation services can choose (in some cases must choose) from available options, so they do.

This is not because lesbians are particularly interested in practicing human engineering. Rather, it seems more related to the culture of consumerism that most of the liquid classes in the United States are more or less comfortable with. Women of the liquid classes know about shopping. They know about cost and quality comparisons. They know about catalogues and secure web-servers. They also know the difference between a sperm donor who sounds "really cute" (e.g., black hair and blue eyes) and one who they are "not interested in" (e.g., the "wrong" ethnicities, with the darkest being the least often chosen).[27] In this shopping mode, the differences between socio-political categories such as race and aesthetic categories (which also have socio-political implications) get leveled by being marketed as equivalent "choices."

Lesbian-oriented infertility services operate with awareness of the range of issues relevant to inseminating lesbians. They advertise themselves as providing a sensitive and caring atmosphere, being lesbian friendly, and being supportive of alternative families. To these ends, they provide a range of services and amenities that aim to facilitate lesbian parenting, not just insemination. Support groups for inseminators, non-biological co-mothers, single lesbians, and interracial lesbian couples; workshops on insemination decision-making; informational orientations and workshops; play groups; literature; and counseling, are among the plethora of social services offered to lesbians at these centers/clinics. These clinics also provide information on legal issues, as well as contacts for legal services, staffed by attorneys experienced in petitioning for second-parent adoption, drawing up donor-contracts, and other intentional lesbian family legal issues. One lesbian-oriented program describes itself as follows:

> Today we continue to provide medical alternatives for achieving conception, as well as a support network, education, and advocacy.

Resources include individual counseling and support groups for women and men considering alternative insemination, adoption, or foster care; medical services and support for women and couples in all stages of the alternative insemination (AI) process; and workshops and discussion groups that address the personal, social, legal, and political issues facing gay/lesbian families.[28]

This kind of holistic approach is markedly different from the biomedicalized experiences lesbians have in the mainstream infertility establishment.

Even the company logos for the lesbian-oriented infertility services have a hip, queer feel to them, consistent with the aesthetic of the community. My favorite on this front is Pacific Reproductive Services (www .hellobaby.com), whose logo is a cute, cartoon, purple ink drawing of a smiling diapered baby and, only slightly smaller than the baby, purple outlines of spermatozoa, all floating on a lavender background. Above the graphic, in big welcoming letters, is PRS's motto, "Hello Baby!" This is a stark contrast to the pastel sentimentality (e.g., "Join the Cycle of Life") and the "übersemen" masculinity (Zygen Laboratories 1997) typically used to represent infertility services.

While most semen bank websites have links to sites such as the American Society for Reproductive Medicine and the American Association of Tissue Banks (AATB), lesbian-oriented infertility services websites typically have links to other sites of relevance to inseminating lesbians. These include the Lesbian Moms' Support Group, Children of Lesbians and Gays Everywhere (COLAGE), The National Center for Lesbian Rights (NCLR), The International Gay and Lesbian Parenting Association (IGLPA), and the Conception Connection. These providers are involved in a project larger than the provision of sperm or the procurement of profit. Indeed, they are part of an infrastructure that supports not just intentional lesbian families, but lesbian culture and survival.

Some interesting comparisons have been drawn between the attitudes of lesbian parents and heterosexual parents in AI families. The evidence so far suggests that lesbians are more concerned than their heterosexual counterparts about the possible deleterious effects of an unknown donor on their children, and much more likely than heterosexual parents to tell the children of their origins in AI.[29] Perhaps because an unplanned pregnancy resulting from a chance encounter is even more stigmatized than a planned lesbian pregnancy, lesbians are virtually unanimous in informing their children of their AI origins. Since lesbians do not have the option that heterosexual parents have of pretending that their child was conceived through conjugal sex, they might tend to give more thought to what to tell the child, and hence how such information might affect the child.

Lesbians, unlike heterosexual women, do not have to consider the feelings of a male partner who may have his own strong reasons for wanting to conceal the insemination. Nor do they have to be concerned to protect the feelings of a social father, whose infertility is generally an emotionally distressing issue that the AI offers to banish from consciousness. Heterosexual women are more ambivalent than lesbians about the process of AI with donor (non-husband) sperm, more likely to consider adoption, and more likely to opt for both secrecy and anonymity.[30]

The men who are married to inseminating women—those who will become the legal and social fathers—are the least inclined of any group to want to tell their future children about their conception. Perhaps because the insemination process represents the loss of a conventionally important part of fatherhood, the social fathers-to-be are also more likely than either inseminating heterosexual or lesbian women to support mandatory counseling for prospective AI parents.[31] And finally, the lesbian partners of inseminating women—the nonbiological co-mothers-to-be—are more likely to want to use semen from "unregistered" (anonymous) donors than their biological-mother partners.[32] This preference may be due to the non-biological mother's legal insecurity regarding her child, or because a known donor represents a threat to her status as second parent, or both.

Because the sperm donor is not a substitute for a male partner, lesbians are understandably less threatened than heterosexual women about disclosing their use of AI to their children and others.[33] Still, as long as women lose custody of their children for being lesbian, many women will opt for anonymous donors to protect their families and limit the chances of intrusion by the donor. Mindful of this and other practical and personal considerations, most lesbian-oriented infertility services also offer anonymous donors, but still provide more information about them. Sperm banks may, for additional fees, offer hand-written letters by the donor to the child-to-be, baby pictures or current pictures, recorded messages, and/or "long-form" questionnaires. One bank (California Cryobank) offers its clients a hand-written, fifteen-page-long letter from the anonymous donor to his future offspring about why he became a donor.

As we have seen in the section on the children's donor concept, purchasing these options may one day satisfy the curiosity or otherwise meet the emotional needs of the child, as well as the mother(s). Unfortunately, it is impossible to tell beforehand what particular piece of information or level of contact a particular child will desire. The question of fathers, and what to tell the children about them, is one that all inseminating lesbians have to face at some point. In a society where the cultural norm (though not the material reality) is still the nuclear family, the child conceived with AI may or may not accept the negation of the category of the meaningful father in her or his life.

Some mothers minimize the role of the donor, instead focusing on the lesbian family, and when necessary, on the semen.[34] In other contexts, such a minimizing gesture easily could be read as dehumanizing to the donor, and perhaps as "cheapening" procreation, babies, and hence life in general. In fact, this objection is at the heart of many feminist (and other) bioethicists' disapproval of contractual and technological procreation.[35] The separation of people, mostly women, into commodified sexual and procreative parts, and the exchange thereof on the open market, is understood to be dehumanizing. In the context of lesbian AI, however, these concerns are mitigated by the continuous bodily integrity of women (and men) in AI. The issues are also greatly complicated by the context of heterosexism and the historical difficulties of lesbians, as women and as "gays," to gain familial autonomy, legitimation, and rights.

Based on both my research and my personal experiences, I have serious reservations about "closed" semen donation (in which the donor remains completely anonymous and unknown forever). The evidence indicating that many children whose genitors are anonymous are disturbed by that fact suggests that we should work to change the circumstances, including the legal vulnerability of lesbian mothers, which necessitate such anonymity.[36] These circumstances pressure inseminating lesbians to choose among less-than-ideal options, often opting for anonymous donor semen over that of a known donor who could later pose a threat to the family. Men who are unwilling to have any contact with their offspring probably have no business intentionally bringing them into the world.

I agree with those who believe it is more important for a child conceived with AI (regardless of the sexual orientation of her parents) to have access to information about the identity of both of her biological parents should she want it than for donors to enjoy complete anonymity.[37] Since the sperm donor has a choice to sell, but the child does not have the choice of how to be conceived, the child's (potential) needs should take precedence.

Of course, it is impossible to know what an individual's best interests will be before he or she is even conceived. In addition to differences between individuals, even between siblings in the same family, people's needs and feelings (interests) change over the life course as they move from a fetus to a baby to a child to an adult.[38] Sociologist Erica Haimes argues that these "interests" are represented in differing ways depending on the stage of life (or pre-life) being assumed.

> Representations of the person conceived have to some extent overlapped and have also gone through various changes: for example, from baby/child (in terms of the success of conception) to child/teenager (in terms of the need for "roots") to child (in terms of welfare needs) to the fetus (in terms of genetic risks) to baby/child (in terms of concerns with development).[39]

Thus "the best interests of the child" standard is limited to the extent that it claims to be a one-size-fits-all solution.

Agreeing to identity and personal information revelation when the child reaches adolescence (say between thirteen and sixteen years of age), if she or he desires it, seems to me a fair compromise of the potential needs of the child(ren), parents, and bio-dads over the course of their lives. I am sympathetic toward the argument for completely open semen donation, but given the socio-legal positions of lesbians in society, such a requirement would bar too many lesbians from becoming mothers. Requiring a registry with identifying information for the offspring to access if she chooses seems like a better protection for all family members involved.

Some have argued that banning anonymous donors would cause a drastic reduction in available sperm and thus make insemination more difficult. And indeed, some studies support this concern. For instance, a 1995 study of fifty-five sperm donors in Great Britain found that 89 percent of the respondents required anonymity to participate.[40] However, this fear of a sperm donor shortage should be laid to rest by the situation in Sweden, where sperm donors must register identifying information that becomes available to their offspring. Despite an initial dip in donor availability after the legislation passed in the early 1990s, the supply rebounded, and there continue to be plenty of willing donors.[41] The Swedish situation supports the data showing that in countries around the world a significant minority, and sometimes a majority, of donors would contribute even if their identity were to be disclosed. I strongly suspect that if sperm banks accept only sperm donors agreeable to identity revelation when the child reaches adolescence, there will still be a good group of sperm from which to choose. Such a self-selection process among donors could also discourage sperm donors from concealing their medical histories for financial gain, and it could discourage multiple donations by "career" sperm donors.

Lesbians for and against AI

Lesbian AI participates in, and constitutes a stand for, intimacy and embodied kinship, without calling for a "return" to an idealized or naturalized patriarchal family. This stand is particularly relevant to ongoing transnational political struggles for hegemony over "the family."[42] These struggles take place in an historical period when we are experiencing both the apparent demotion (the much-heralded "breakdown") of the nuclear family and its nostalgic resurrection. Nostalgia for a state of "nature," however, is problematic for lesbians, who have long been considered unnatural.[43]

Therefore, lesbian AI decenters the presumably heterosexual family, including its sexist and heterosexist foundational dualisms, and disputes its claim to be all that is. When a lesbian couple has a baby with the help of AI, for instance, who is inside the family and who outside? Is the arrangement, and the resulting child, "legitimate" or "illegitimate"? What happens to the boundaries between biology and technology, stranger and kin, natural and unnatural? (Mis)understandings of the lesbian (bad, failed, masculine, or non-woman) and the mother (good, married, feminine, or real woman) as polar opposites are challenged.

Families formed with the help of AI are similar to, but not identical to, other family forms. The similarities—that is, somebody has got to do the dishes, comfort the crying child, go to parent-teacher meetings—are often overlooked by those who choose to see the lesbian parents as simply "sex partners." Lesbian mothers often emphasize these similarities in order to gain acceptance for themselves and their families. However, intentional lesbian families are also unique, and their distinctive characteristics deserve mention as well.

Some of the issues that contextualize lesbian discourse about AI include AI versus adoption, using known versus unknown sperm donors, the mother and child's relationship to the genitor if he is known, legal issues around custody, how to self-inseminate, and what to tell the children and when.[44] Also pervading this discourse are practical discussions of loving and raising children in unconventional kinship arrangements.[45] Issues about how to provide bonding, support, and role models for children are taken up, as are ways of ensuring meaningful adult male participation in the lives of sons and daughters. Much of this discourse amounts to nothing less than a radical revisioning of kinship and family for the post-heteropatriarchal, ultramodern family.

This explosion of imaginative attention to lesbian kinship is typified by the 1987 anthology *Politics of the Heart*. In it, numerous lesbians write "from the heart" about their struggles, triumphs, pleasures, and pains in families. Most pieces are autobiographical. Some are scholarly. These essays take the reader on a sojourn through the "uncharted territory" of lesbian motherhood. *Politics of the Heart* introduces the reader not only to the many ways of being a lesbian mother, but also to lesbians who chose not to have children, lesbians who relinquished custody of their children, pseudonymous lesbians who are in the closet and write about it, and lesbian mothers whose children were born within previous heterosexual unions. Yet rather than becoming a parody of inclusiveness by attempting to "cover all the bases," this anthology gains its strength from the true heterogeneity of voices between its covers, and from the topical and substantive depth and richness it brings to lesbian family discourse. Thus the culture that lesbians are creating around their families is not easily assimilated into pre-formed discourses of kinship and motherhood. It problematizes issues that are naturalized and invisible within conventional heteropatriarchal contexts, and participates in the heterogeneity that characterizes postmodern families.

Regarding the lesbian baby boom, some lesbians argue that the prevalence of lesbian mothering is a reactionary trend, a retreat from lesbian-feminist politics, and even a development that has the potential to divide the lesbian community and further marginalize all women without children.[46] If the feminine imperative to be a mother expands to include lesbians, then lesbians would experience increasing social pressure to mother, which is not exactly a liberating prospect. Many lesbian mothers experience alienation from their former social circles or communities when they have children.[47] Of course, heterosexual new parents may also feel alienated from their childless friends. In a heterosexist world, however, becoming alienated from one's community can be a more serious loss for lesbians.

Pro-mother lesbians span the political spectrum. On the one end, lesbian mothering is held out as a radical, avant-garde political activity, perhaps the equivalent of holding a mid-sized gay rights demonstration every day of the child's life.[48] In the middle are the more "liberal" arguments about lesbian rights to motherhood and marriage—and divorce.[49] Conservative arguments for same-sex marriage (including parenting) are also in circulation.[50] Wherever they may be on this latter spectrum, intentional lesbian mothers challenge the dominant nostalgic paradigms of family, motherhood, and womanhood in ways that create more space for all of us.

The Lesbian Mother Closet

One of the many ways that AI motherhood affects lesbians is how it changes their relationship to the closet and "outness." Some women find that becoming mothers, and having children, makes their lesbian identities less visible, as they are seen as "mothers" first, and their lesbian identity is eclipsed by their maternal identity. They may (or may not) be less targeted for heterosexist harassment and assault, but feel "re-closeted."

This can be especially distressing if it happens in front of the child(ren). The NLFS found that such instances of "mistaken assumptions of heterosexuality" were common occurrences for the mothers, and that 25 percent of the mothers reported feeling "quite distressed" when their child witnessed such heterosexism.[51]

Other lesbians, or the same lesbians at different times, feel that insemination and motherhood "outs" them as lesbians as never before. The persistent "innocent" (heteronormative) question about the child's father forces a reckoning with the fact of a woman's lesbian identity. She is compelled in that instant either to lie—make up a story about the "father"—or to come out and tell the innocent questioner some or all of the truth: that she is a lesbian, that the child's other parent is her woman lover, and/or that the child was conceived through AI. As lesbian mothers wind their ways through the multiple institutional contexts of parenting   pediatricians, other mothers at the playground, child care, teachers and PTAs, birthday parties, dealings with the welfare state, religious training—they face "innocent" questions demanding a revelation of lesbian identity, or its concealment.[52] Many lesbian mothers have written of the stresses and joys of coming out in such random, daily, "innocent" situations.[53]

In this context, lesbian identity is about kinship at least as much as it is about sexuality. Questions about kinship—who is the father, who is the mother, does she have any brothers or sisters, does she take after her father—demand answers that reveal lesbian identity. Keeping one's lesbian identity secret becomes less plausible when children are involved, since questions of kinship can no longer be avoided, as they might be before one is pregnant or has children, when a lesbian can "simply" avoid discussing her "personal" life.

This blurry line between sexuality and kinship is at the heart of ignorance about lesbian existence. Weston discusses the slippages between kinship talk and sexuality talk in *Families We Choose* (1991). She explains how lesbian and gay talk about kinship—one's partner/lover, one's children, holiday plans, whether a child is sick, who comes to the parent-teacher conference—is interpreted homophobically as inappropriate talk about sexuality. The paradoxical bind is that lesbians who may have absolutely no wish to talk about their sexuality are accused of exactly that when they talk about their families. Ironically, it is the heterosexist listener, who says "what you do in your bedroom is your business, just don't flaunt it in my face," who insists on viewing all things lesbian as sexual.

In the context of lesbian motherhood, "coming out" is as much a declaration of kinship status as it is of sexual identity. This is particularly true of lesbians who have children in a lesbian relationship or community, rather than those lesbians who had children in a previous heterosexual relationship and came out later (and who can more easily hide behind the less-stigmatized label "single mother"). Of course, single lesbian mothers can hide this way as well. Lesbians also use invisibility strategically. Since most lesbians are assumed to be heterosexual by virtue of being human, they have to, and get to, decide when, where, and to whom to come out as lesbians. Lesbian psychotherapist and author JoAnn Loulan believes that every lesbian has a Rolodex in her mind where she keeps track of who she's come out to and to what degree.[54] While this is emotionally taxing, it also provides opportunities to work strategically with invisibility. On the most obvious level, when dealing with homophobic doctors, one might choose not to disclose her lesbian identity. On a more subtle level, someone may choose to use her clothes, mannerisms, and even subtle flirting behavior to promote an image of herself as heterosexual in certain situations. The NLFS found that of the 85 percent of lesbian moms who were mistakenly assumed to be heterosexual, 21 percent of them "liked 'fitting in more' as a result of that assumption."[55] There are costs to this, as in any closeted situation, but invisibility can allow some people options that they would not otherwise have if everyone knew they were lesbian.

Blood Ties and Chosen Kin

The issue of "blood ties" arises when we talk about gay family, and particularly about lesbian mothering. Lesbians, along with gay men, are equated in the popular imagination with loneliness, excessive sexuality, and lack of family. In part due to lesbians' (and gay men's) exclusion from legal, religious, medico-psychiatric, and social legitimation for their families, and in part due to rejection by families of origin upon coming out, lesbians (like other stigmatized groups) have created unique and ingenious kinship forms to meet their needs.[56] These relationships most often include relationships of primary importance that have no biogenetic or legal basis. A person's lover, ex-lovers, gay male friends, important children in their lives, non-rejecting "blood" kin, and even companion animals, may all be part of a lesbian's family. This circle of kin of course varies across class, ethnicity, race, "outness," region, and many other axes.

Kath Weston, an anthropologist working in the San Francisco Bay Area, found that lesbians and gay men tend to articulate their families in two distinct categories: blood or straight family, and chosen or gay family.[57] These LGBT-defined categories draw from the same discursive resources as others do, including the various tropes of feudal and modern families. According to Weston, the dominant metaphors of gay family, especially for women, are choice, "freedom from," will, liberation, and options. These categories contrast to their opposites attributed to "straight family," including blood and genes, non-choice, heterosexuality, heterosexism and "straight" marriage.

The prevalence of these categories, "families we choose" versus "blood families," is far from random. They reflect the autonomy and courage needed to come out of the closet. Through this distinction, the two kinds of family are leveled, though not collapsed. Important symbolic operations are effected in this (queer) kinship discourse.

One is that "blood" family is both remystified and demystified. It is remystified through the continued articulation of one's family of origin as being on the natural and biological side of a conventional Western metaphysical split. By not challenging the "naturalness" of "blood" family, and continuing to use naturalized metaphors for it, lesbians and gay men remain within the conventional discourse that pits nature against will or "choice."[58] In the process, the presumed heterosexuality and "blood ties" of families of origin are unwittingly reinforced. Since only some children are raised by relatives to whom they have genetic or "blood" ties, and virtually all of us have some lesbian, gay, or bisexual members in our families of origin, to call those families "straight" discursively erases our nonheterosexual relatives and thus enforces lesbian invisibility. To call those families "blood" erases the choice involved in their construction.

Yet many lesbians and gay men demystify hegemonic and nostalgic expectations of family (e.g., as loving, constant, protective, natural, unbreakable ties) simply by being gay. A lesbian who contemplates coming out to her "straight" family is well aware that the outcome of such a revelation is unpredictable, no matter how certain she feels about how people will react. Even if "blood" family members react in the best possible way, with instantaneous and absolute loving support, the lesbian will not have been spared the frightening experience of contemplating the possible and prevalent negative outcomes that are frequently detailed in lesbian and gay discourse. By going through the coming-out process, a lesbian or gay man faces the fact that "blood" ties are not inviolable, but are chosen perhaps as much as gay relationships. This demystification, even if it goes on below the conscious level, serves to strengthen ties to one's chosen family, whose realness as family is reinforced.[59]

It is difficult to estimate the longevity of lesbian relationships for the same reason that it is difficult to estimate almost anything about how lesbians live: few researchers are asking, so we have little solid data. In the conservative climate in Washington, studies that research and document lesbian realities do not get funded. This is partly because of heterosexism, and partly because studies of lesbians are seen as "sex studies," which can rarely get funding, even to find out what heterosexual married couples are doing in bed.

A major study done in the early 1980s, before the lesbian baby boom, found that lesbian relationships are shorter-lived than either gay male or heterosexual pairings. However, newer research has found little if any difference in the longevity of lesbian and other types of relationships. The NLFS found lesbian relationships lasting as long as heterosexual relationships. As the NLFS reports:

> Recent estimates suggest that over one-half of all children born to heterosexual parents will experience marital disruption. Data from the NLFS suggest a comparable divorce rate among lesbian mothers. [Citations omitted.][60]

While the data is not sufficient to draw any solid conclusions, we at least have reason not to assume the worst about lesbian relationship longevity, particularly when children are involved.

At the same time that "blood" ties are devalorized, the practice of lesbian AI reintroduces biology into the "gay" family. While lesbians and gay men debate the ramifications of this development, it appears to be largely lauded as positive, and many see AI babies as icons of the lesbian community. Particularly early in the lesbian baby boom, a sense of collective celebration ensued when two women became parents together.

Kath Weston argues that the queer construct "families we choose" undermines the conventional wisdom that asserts that straight is to gay as family is to no family.[61] Instead, Weston documents how lesbians and gay men construct their kinship networks as "chosen" families, an act that disrupts the discourse that puts gays outside the realm of kinship. With "gay family," Weston argues, lesbians and gay men break the binary opposition between the heterosexual family and the homosexual non-family, and instead invent a third category, "gay family," which enables lesbians and gay men to both be queer and have family.

This creation of a third term reflects not only a different kind of (postmodern) family, but also a different (postmodern) way of thinking about family than those of feudal or modern family discourses. Lesbian and gay families, as Weston argues, are not merely derivative or substitutive of "normal" families, but constitute a historical development of kinship in the 1980s and beyond. Through discursive and material reframing, intentional lesbian families exemplify Stacey's "postmodern family."

> No longer is there a single culturally dominant family pattern, like the "modern" one, to which a majority of citizens conform and most of the rest aspire. Instead, postindustrial conditions have compelled and encouraged us to craft a wide array of family arrangements, which we inhabit uneasily and reconstitute frequently as our occupational and personal circumstances shift.[62]

Liberatory, transgressive, regressive, anti-homophobic, privatized, like and unlike nuclear and extended families, pronatalist, technological and biological, maternalist and anti-patriarchal, para-parthenogenic: Intentional lesbian families could not possibly be more "postmodern."

In Iowa, Petra and Adrienne received a tremendous welcome from the gay and lesbian community when their daughter, Kim, was born. Petra describes,

> "There were lots of lesbian mothers around who had been married, but no other parents "by choice" nearby. We were quite aware that we were forging new ground. Plus we were both pretty public figures in the

professional community. All other lesbians in town go to Adrienne for their gynecologic care, and many of my clients are lesbians, so it became a community event. It's like Kim is the community's baby . . . People seemed to lock onto this as some affirmation of their existence and a validation of life, and it was just overwhelming."[63]

Even in those areas of the country where intentional lesbian motherhood is no longer a groundbreaking event, many lesbians find it affirming to see other lesbians having babies. As Judith Stacey argues, all families now partake of the contingent, unstable, and diverse quality of postmodernity. Since this condition is most visible in "queer" families, they serve as a lightning rod for cultural anxieties about family change.[64]

Radical or Conservative?

At the same time that lesbian AI can be radical, transgressive, and challenging to the status quo, it reinforces dominant sex, gender, and class norms in important ways. I have discussed some ways that lesbian families share with heterosexuals the dominant class–based values about what makes a family in terms of wealth.

Scholars and other observers disagree about whether lesbian-mother families reinforce or challenge gender roles. Sociologist Maureen Sullivan has observed that, in lesbian households, the division of labor is not determined by the sex of the partner, so gender norms are being challenged.[65] Since biological sex cannot determine who does what, either in the work force or around the home, and since many lesbian couples place a strong positive value on equality and negotiation of roles and responsibilities, these lesbian-mother families are in effect "undoing gender." At the same time, not all lesbian-mother families are as egalitarian as they would like to believe, and as they may seem to others.

Sullivan studied thirty-four Northern California lesbian co-parent families, most, if not all, of which had used AI. Among them, she found two distinct arrangements. She found that "equitable practices—a pattern of equal sharing" was the norm. She noted, however, that a minority of families had a primary breadwinner/primary caretaker division of labor. In these "Rozzie and Harriet" families, Sullivan found that the partner with the role of primary caretaker experienced disempowerment, dissatisfaction, and loss of self-esteem similar to what heterosexual women experience in that role. She concludes that the financial dependence in such an unequal division of domestic labor takes a serious toll on the dependent partner, independent of gender.[66]

Christopher Carrington has an even less sanguine view. Based on his study of twenty-six lesbian families and twenty-six gay male families, he concludes that:

> Lesbigay family members desire perfect order and meaningful patterns, both in material and in emotional terms. For better or for worse, the ideals lesbigay families aspire to attain are often quite similar to those of their heterosexual peers.[67]

Most lesbian (and gay male) couples were not particularly egalitarian. Rather, he found these couples emotionally and politically invested in believing that they were egalitarian, and in presenting themselves as such to the world. While he did find the lesbian families to be more egalitarian than the male ones, he found family members continually trying to manage inequalities between them. Through close observation, including living with some of his subjects for a week at a time, and by asking much more detailed questions about "invisible" domestic work than is typical, a striking picture emerged.

> "[P]artners in many lesbigay relationships work together to camouflage the actual divisions of domesticity and to prevent threats to the gender identities of their partners, particularly for women who do little domestic work and for men who do a lot."[68]

Coupled lesbians, in other words, would deny inequalities between them, and assert that both were equally "feminine." Interestingly, the families he studied disavowed butch/femme divisions of domestic labor, when in Carrington's observations, many of their domestic arrangements were more akin to the butch/femme arrangements of the 1950s than to the egalitarian ideals they espoused.[69]

Those couples that came closest to achieving the longed-for equality were those at the top of the class structure. They "bought" equality in their relationships by hiring out domestic work to underpaid housecleaners, gardeners, launderers, caterers, and (I would add) nannies. In their efforts not to exploit one member of the couple, Carrington asserted, wealthier lesbian and gay families instead exploited workers outside the family, a problematic solution at best.[70]

Many lesbians are still struggling to figure out how to share their lives equitably and without exploitation, so that their family members can thrive. Without recognizing the difficulties in achieving such equality, however, we are less likely to attain it. I know this is true in my own relationship with my partner, who is our young son's stay-at-home daddy. Carrington summarizes,

> Those who would place lesbigay families on the egalitarian pedestal need to come to terms with the fragility of lesbigay relationships. Fully aware of this fragility, many lesbigay family members who might invest more energy in domesticity probably do not, instead putting more energy into paid work and consequently reducing the quality and the long-term durability of their family relationships.[71]

In other words, we—and here I'm not just talking about lesbians, but about diverse families at this point in history—do not trust that our relationships will last, and so we do not want to invest domestically (and possibly emotionally) in something that may not be there in a couple of years. The Catch-22 is that when we do not invest as fully as we might, our relationships are less likely to survive and thrive.

Most families, regardless of gender or sexual orientation, face formidable barriers to equality, longevity, and happiness. It may well be that most lesbian families are egalitarian, as Sullivan found, particularly when compared to heterosexual ones. The complex issues involved, and the contradictory findings of researchers on this issue, however, should help to insulate us from platitudes that paint heterosexuality, or men, as the sole sources of inequality in families.

7

Conclusions
Toward a Lesbian-Normative Universe and AI Family Futures

ABSTRACT

In this chapter, I review approaches to change that have been proposed to improve the conditions of inseminating lesbians and their families. I emphasize legal changes, but discuss philosophical, institutional, and interpersonal approaches as well. I conclude with an attempt to envision a lesbian-normative universe.

Approaches to Change

Since the situation of inseminating lesbians and their families is inseparable from larger cultural, institutional, and discursive processes, revolutionary changes may be necessary to improve their situation. Full citizenship and self-determination for lesbians, including the right of lesbians (and other women) to raise their families without men if they so wish, basic human rights guarantees (e.g., food, shelter, health care, freedom of association), and expanded social justice are some changes necessary to true empowerment of intentional lesbian family members. Given that lesbians are a diverse population, providing full human rights to all of them means raising the level of existence for the least empowered as well as those with the most resources and privilege. Such revolutionary changes will probably continue to occur incrementally, with backlash an omnipresent challenge to each advance, however small. In addition to such sweeping changes, more circumscribed policy reforms are needed.

To improve the legal situation of intentional lesbian families, we need to work on many fronts—from the macro to the micro, in legal, political, interpersonal, and cultural arenas. Legal reform alone, while crucial, is inadequate. It also would be foolish to privilege utopian and radical reform (e.g., abolishing marriage as a legal category), which has little practical chance of being enacted, even if it might be the best option. Neither should we dismiss the importance of less ambitious incremental reforms (e.g., working for domestic-partner benefits at one's workplace) that may benefit people significantly, even if they are profoundly partial.

What follow are some of the most promising approaches to the problems described thus far. By studying this wide array, we gain a picture of the proliferation of resistance that accompanies the proliferation of oppression against inseminating lesbians and their families. As legal scholar Robin West writes,

> Perhaps the greatest obstacle to the creation of a feminist jurisprudence is that feminist jurisprudence must simultaneously confront both political and conceptual barriers to women's freedom. The political barrier is surely the most pressing. Feminists must first and foremost counter a profound power imbalance, and the way to do that is through law and politics.[1]

Resistance takes place, of course, within the framework of highly politicized and ideological discourses on "the family." Lesbian scholars and activists do not have the alternative of waxing nostalgic for an idealized and naturalized family along the "Leave it to Beaver" model. Their approaches span the liberal to radical spectrum. An ironic and sometimes surprising effect is that those strategies most easily defined as "liberal"—working within the system—often have the most wide-ranging and "radical" effects both institutionally and ideologically. Those approaches most identifiable as "radical"—calling for an overhaul of the underlying tenets of the system as well as its operations—are often too "far out" to make much impact. It is a sad comment on the state of lesbian rights that even the most basic civil liberties must still be fought for aggressively, and simply overturning the laws that make lesbian sexual expressions illegal is major progress.

Changing the System from Within

Lesbians pursue case-by-case challenges of existing laws, drawing on precedents set for other family structures and stretching them to fit the needs of intentional lesbian families. If they are successful, they help set new legal precedents that may benefit others as well. Claims by nonbiological lesbian mothers to de facto parental status or to standing as *in loco parentis* have been widespread, both in the fight for second-parent adoption, and in visitation battles after a breakup. Lesbian mothers have used equitable estoppel to protect their family from intrusion by a sperm donor.[2]

It is possible that U.S. lesbians who are discriminated against by AI providers (physicians, hospitals, sperm banks) could use public accommodations laws. Lesbians in British Columbia, Canada, have successfully done so. Legal scholar Holly Harlow argues for this use of public accommodations laws and points to the precedent set by a group of pregnant women in New York who won the right to be treated in a hospital-based detoxification program that originally refused to treat any pregnant women.[3] She points out that while most physician discrimination against "single women" (a category in which she explicitly includes lesbians) is based on personal, religious, or philosophical beliefs and "beyond the reach of constitutional challenge," hospitals employing such physicians may be successfully challenged.

These types of approaches, which work within existing legal parameters to win, are important and legitimate. The court system should provide justice to lesbian mothers and their families.

Changing or Overturning Existing Laws and Creating New Laws

Because no state has yet recognized or honored same-sex marriage, gay men and lesbians have sought legal protections for their relationships and families through other routes. Domestic-partnership benefits, power-of-attorney agreements, anti-discrimination statutes, civil union legislation, and second-parent adoption have each afforded important protections. In addition to working with existing laws, lesbians pursue statutory and legislative challenges to laws that unfairly disadvantage them and their families.

A highly publicized movement to legalize same-sex marriage (and a backlash against that movement) began in the 1990s. Efforts to overturn the ban on lesbians and gay men serving openly in the U.S. military have been similarly publicized. Overturning sodomy laws, pursuing domestic-partnership legislation, and organizing for civil rights laws to protect lesbians and their families are other instances in which the laws themselves are recognized to be inadequate. Such struggles have had important impacts on the lives of inseminating lesbians and their families. For instance, the overturning of sodomy laws by the U.S. Supreme Court has had a sometimes subtle, sometimes dramatic, but in any case significant, effect on the lives of lesbians and their families.

Though some find the symbolics of marriage offensive, the legalization of lesbian marriage may be the farthest-reaching way to grant legal equality to lesbian families. The denial of marriage to lesbians is a blatant and intolerable form of sex discrimination that contributes to the marginalization and oppression of lesbians and their families. Lack of access to marriage confers on lesbians (and gay men) the legal status of children and "the mentally incompetent." While granting a basic human right, changing the laws to allow lesbians to marry would solve many legal problems of lesbian AI in one fell swoop.

Such a change would grant parental status for lesbian co-mothers under existing laws. A co-mother by marriage would automatically be treated as legal parent regarding housing, immigration, welfare, insurance, custody and visitation, rights of intestate succession, hospital and prison visitation, school participation, and other essential issues. Marriage would protect both mothers from intrusion by the sperm donor in states where that right is given to married women. (Of course, such a statute should be implemented in states where it is not already on the books.) Since the advent of Civil Union law, these benefits and responsibilities of marriage (except for immigration) are now officially available to same-sex couples in the state of Vermont. Legalizing same-sex marriage would enhance the security, continuity, and psychological well-being of children of such unions.[4] Legalization would create the social expectation that nonbiological lesbian parents be responsible to their children, since their obligations would be the same as those of the adoptive or biological parents in any divorce.[5]

The legal system needs to reinforce these changes by banning discrimination based on sexual orientation, sex, or marital status. Universal, non-homophobic health insurance would provide medicalized AI to those who want it, without regard to wealth. Generous welfare state guarantees (e.g., housing, health care, poverty relief) would prevent any woman from having to depend on the largesse of individual fathers to provide for their children. It would also facilitate the transformation of the legal definition of families into a more flexible category that better meets today's needs.

Feminist Reforms of the Family

Lesbians have benefited from strategies that emphasize women's rights in the family. It bears stating that in addition to being oppressed for being "queer," lesbian mothers are also disadvantaged as women. As the legal position of mothers is strengthened, the legal position of lesbian mothers is strengthened. As feminists in the international human rights movement so aptly state, "Women's Rights Are Human Rights." Lesbian human rights activists have elaborated on this slogan: "Lesbian Rights Are Women's Rights. Women's Rights Are Human Rights. Lesbian Rights Are Human Rights." Rachel Rosenbloom continues,

> Women's rights and lesbian rights are linked in substantive ways. Both issues challenge how human rights distinctions between the private and public and reluctance to address female sexuality have perpetuated violations of women and kept them invisible. The defense of lesbian rights is integral to the defense of all women's right to determine their own sexuality, to work at the jobs they prefer, and to live as they choose with women, men, children, or alone. Heterosexism and fear of lesbianism is used to keep women in line —accepting their society's assigned gender roles and limitations. When any woman curtails her freedom or fails to take an action or say what she believes out of fear of being labeled a lesbian, then heterosexism has denied her independence and sapped her strength.[6]

So, when the right of women to live and parent autonomously from men is safeguarded, the right of lesbians to live and raise their children is protected too. The reverse is also true.

This connection between women's rights and lesbian rights may seem so evident as to require no elaboration, but the insidious divide-and-conquer effects of heterosexism threaten to disguise this point at every turn. Critics of the "lesbians as women" approach, however, point out that heterosexual women's needs and experiences are not necessarily the same as those of lesbians. Because lesbians face oppression as lesbians, a specifically lesbian jurisprudence—and a specifically lesbian liberation movement—is needed. Lesbian jurisprudence, while feminist and gay, prioritizes lesbian legal issues ahead of those of other constituencies, thus clarifying and foregrounding how lesbian existence is unique. Such jurisprudence has no conflict of interest and no confusion when an intentional lesbian family is pitted against a gay male sperm donor.[7] The development of a specifically lesbian jurisprudence (as opposed to a gay and lesbian jurisprudence) is still at such an early stage that it is impossible to know what it will look like in even ten years. I hope and expect for it to develop as an important supplement and counterpoint to feminist jurisprudence and gay and lesbian jurisprudence, particularly in regard to lesbian-centered issues such as AI kinship.

Changing the (Non-Legal) Rules

The pursuit of changes in social institutions other than the law are also important. Changes in the U.S. workplace to minimize discrimination against and disadvantaging of lesbians are a salient example. Lesbians and their allies have won same-sex domestic partnership benefits in health care, personal/family leave, and other benefits in several hundred companies across the United States. While most lesbians do not work in these companies, such a progressive stance sets a tone that affects the climate of the larger world of work.

Other important non-legal approaches include adding sexual orientation to the non-discrimination policies of public and private employers, and such basic victories as allowing lesbian families to qualify for "married student housing" on university campuses. As the health insurance industry increases its power in the medical system, non-discriminatory insurance policies become increasingly important.

Changing Lesbian Culture, Attitudes, and Behavior

Lesbians also privately and publicly exhort each other to personal responsibility and honor regarding family ethics. These calls range from the practical to the absurd. On the useful side of the spectrum, the National Center for Lesbian Rights (NCLR) held a series of fora for the lesbian community and for lesbian-rights attorneys to discuss the then-new phenomenon of lesbians bringing each other to court after a breakup.

The NCLR sought to develop a dialogue within the lesbian community about lesbian family ethics, and to promote alternatives to the legal system for lesbian family dispute resolution. These public discussions were important not only because they may have inspired better behavior by individuals, but also because they educated part of the attorney pool from which lesbian litigants are likely to draw in their battles against each other. As NCLR staff members wrote in "Our Day In Court—Against Each Other: Intra-community Disputes Threaten All of Our Rights," referring to agreements among lesbian family members,

> What do we do when agreements and feelings change? How do we want to define who a parent is? What role should biology play? How do we consider the wishes of our children?
>
> NCLR has been participating in roundtable discussions of these questions with other gay- and lesbian-rights advocates. And we will be sponsoring a series of public forums on some of the current issues arising in intra-community disputes. Without this dialogue and understanding, we will soon find lesbian and gay legal organizations arguing against each other in court, right along with the other members of our community.[8]

While the activities of NCLR in this regard are hardly limited to discussions of "personal responsibility," they broach issues regarding standards of behavior, and aim to envision and promote what is good in and for lesbian families and family members.

On the other hand, some lesbians call for personal responsibility without taking into account the social and political contexts. While this approach receives most of its airtime in the popular gay press and among legal practitioners, it also has its advocates among legal scholars. Lesbian legal scholar Shelley Gavigan typifies this stream, condemning lesbians for taking each other to court, and excoriating both biological and non-biological lesbian mothers alike for denying their children's relationship to the nonbiological parent after a breakup.[9] Others in gay and lesbian communities have used public fora (newspapers, scholarly and popular articles, community meetings) to chastise litigants in such cases.

While community expectations do have an impact on people's behavior, approaches directed at individuals seem the least likely to yield pro-intentional lesbian family results. As is amply demonstrated by the entire corpus of divorce case law, people who are in the midst of "divorce" do not often behave rationally or benevolently toward their ex-mates. To the extent that the law allows lesbian co-mothers to disavow parental relationships with their nonbiological children, some will do so. As long as the law allows lesbian biological mothers to deny the parental status of their children's nonbiological mother, some will do so. These realities have sometimes shocked those in the lesbian community who would like to believe that lesbians are more civilized than others when they end relationships. Still, they are a fact of life.[10]

Unfortunately, those who believe exhortations to "sisterhood" will change behavior among divorcing, custody-battling parents of any orientation are probably wasting their breath. Most of us know that even the impassioned pleas of close friends and family members seldom stem the tide of contentious and adversarial divorce litigation, particularly when children are involved. To suppose that lesbians will be morally "better" than everyone else in this situation is unrealistic and unhelpful. Lesbians will generally use whatever financial, legal, and other resources are available to try to win their cases. That the heterosexism, misogyny, racism, and other forms of oppression structured into the legal system are among these resources is not the fault of the litigants. Neither is it their prerogative to shape the legal context in which they fight. Rather it is the responsibility of the judiciary, the legislature, and the electorate to ensure that such legal options as the denial of the nonbiological mother's parenthood are not available.[11]

Fathers, for example, often deny their parental status in attempts to be free of financial obligations toward offspring. Indeed, much case law relating to AI involves such suits. While they are rarely successful, it is a prevalent enough tactic that all fifty states have statutes protecting children from this male response to the breakup with the children's mother (regardless of his biological link to the children). While the automatic attribution of fatherhood status to male genitors is not unproblematic, such laws could be applied equally to female nonbiological parents who seek to shirk familial obligations.

An Australian court made such a ruling for child support on the part of a nonbiological lesbian co-mother. The 1996 court ordered a lesbian co-mother to pay the equivalent of U.S. $113,000 in "maintenance" to her former partner who is raising their two children conceived with AI. The couple had been together from 1986 to 1994, and the children were born in 1989 and 1992. Supreme Court Judge David Hobson said about the case, "In my opinion it is unconscionable for the defendant now to seek to make no contribution whatsoever to the upbringing of the children."[12]

There have also been U.S. cases where the judge found the lesbian co-mother liable for child support payments. In 2002, a Massachusetts judge ordered a lesbian co-mother to pay child support for both of the ex-couple's children. The co-mother had legally adopted the second child only, and asserted she therefore should not have to help support the other, who was unrelated to her by blood or law. As in the Australian case, the judge chastised the would-be-deadbeat mom, saying that she, as the "major provider of the family unit," had to step up to the plate.[13] Referring to the Massachusetts Supreme Judicial Court ruling that allows visitation and other rights to de facto parents, he said that it "would not make any sense" to offer such privileges without corresponding responsibilities. While it remains to be seen what will happen on appeal, this case is rightly seen as a landmark ruling that supports the normalization of lesbian divorce, and hence lesbian marriage and motherhood. This is the type of "public" exhortation to familial responsibility that is most likely to affect others' future behavior.

Theoretical Approaches to Change: Changing the Definition of Family

Many lesbians and feminists are vigorously debating theoretical and philosophical positions that might underlie the creation of lesbian and/or feminist jurisprudence. A major area of discussion is how to rework existing definitions of the family to better meet the needs of family members. Legal literature provides a dazzling spectrum of opinions as to how current definitions of the family need to change. While reimagining and transforming kinship and family organization are hardly new feminist projects, some of the most creative and visionary theorizing in feminist family scholarship is taking place among legal scholars.[14] I cannot provide a comprehensive overview of this diverse and vital body of work, but I will discuss some approaches that are directly relevant to the issues addressed in this book.

The "Functional" Family

Adopting a "functional" definition of the family, rather than the conventional "formal" definition, is one potential solution for the situation of lesbian AI and other postmodern families. Under a functional definition, such as that pioneered by legal scholar Martha Minow (the attorney in the *Alison M* case), those who act as a family should be treated as one by the law.[15] Minow suggests a "functional" parent might be defined as "someone who has taken care of the child on a daily basis, is known to the child as a parent, and has provided love and financial support." Such a definition of family, she argues, would go a long way toward securing the legal protection of lesbian families. All functional families would be treated equally under the law. Within this framework, Minow advocates "a liberal approach to family membership but a strict view of family obligations."[16] While legal equality for all families would allow people to enter into a variety of family arrangements, there should be few ways of severing ties to dependents. This model, Minow asserts, is not only in the best interest of the children, but of adult family members and society as well.

Critics of the functional approach believe such a change is not enough to protect "alternative" families. Rather than conferring "the same autonomy and stability as traditional families, freedom to choose, and preservation of relationships," the functional approach leaves too much to the discretion of the court.[17] This is a point even proponents of the functional approach are willing to grant.[18] The functional definition of family is charged with being "indeterminate, intrusive, and unfair."[19] This lack of precision, it is argued, denies family members secure knowledge of their legal status, thereby defeating its purpose.[20]

Legally Binding Family Contracts

Instead, some critics of the functional approach argue for a family registration system that would grant registered families, of whatever persuasion, the same legal rights and obligations as those conferred by marriage and adoption. This system of open registration would create "a presumption of legality," and reduce the marginalization of lesbian and other postmodern families.[21]

Legal scholar Vickie Henry promotes one variation on this theme. Henry argues that membership in a family in cases of AI should be determined by a legally binding contract that delineates specific familial relationships, signed by all adult parties (which may include a known donor, a lesbian co-mother, or other "alternative" family members) prior to the birth of the child.[22] This formulation attempts to take some of the uncertainty out of families that are defined functionally rather than biologically or through marriage. In Henry's scheme, all parties would know from day one what their legal roles would be, and the judiciary would be compelled to honor the parameters chosen by that particular family.

This approach is also advocated by the National Center for Lesbian Rights (NCLR). The NCLR, which has vast experience in litigating such cases, urges all participants in the creation of planned lesbian families to draw up legal documents explicating their intentions. While the NCLR acknowledges that such contracts are not legally binding, they have the benefit of clarifying expectations. This means there is less chance of conflict in the future. They also provide documentation that can support legal claims as to the signatories' intended relationships in case they do end up in court. This approach may be particularly appropriate to families formed with the help of contractual or technological procreation such as AI. As the NCLR elaborates,

> Many legal commentators have advocated the intent model [of family definition] since the traditional family law paradigm cannot accommodate the complex issues presented by reproductive technologies. These

scholars argue that only a contract law model can effectively address the competing interests involved. We agree.[23]

Many lesbians who inseminate in fact do just this. Contracts signed by mothers and donor detail what the relationships to the child will be and what will happen in the event of any future dispute.[24] While courts use their discretion to evaluate the best interests of the child, the contract may be one of several factors the court considers. Books and other resources for potential inseminators sometimes include sample contracts for biological mother, co-mother, and sperm donor to encourage their use.[25]

The Value of Care and Rights

This view, however, is far from unanimous among lesbians, feminists, or anyone else. Feminist scholars are divided, or perhaps ambivalent, about contract, and its co-discourses of individualism, private property, free will, and the rule of law. In feminist theorizing, contract has been associated with the gendered division between care and rights that preoccupied Western feminists throughout the 1980s.

A focus on the value of care stems from contemporary research on gender and moral development that supports an alternative to the primacy of the contractual model of human interaction that is reified in modern legal systems.[26] Often stopping short of radically challenging current gender arrangements, these scholars find value-neutral "differences" between typical male and female socialization patterns, and argue for their equal valuation.

According to this body of scholarship (epitomized by Carol Gilligan and sometimes referred to as "difference feminism"), women are socialized to operate from a "morality of care," while men operate from a "morality of rights." In the words of Rand Jack and Dana Crowley Jack,

> [Men] experience society as composed of autonomous, separate individuals. A hierarchy of rules, rights, and obligations mediate human interactions and help preserve independence . . . [R]elationships are conceived in contractual terms and are subject to negotiation . . . [I]ntimacy and interdependence can threaten the right to be free autonomous individuals.[27]

Women, on the other hand tend to be,

> more empathic, caring, service-oriented, relationship oriented, and con-
> cerned with others' feelings. Women judge themselves in terms of their
> ability to care and the feminine personality comes to define itself in rela-
> tion and connection to other people.[28]

These differences set up many opportunities for disappointment and confusion on an interpersonal level, as well as the devaluation of both women
and caring on a macro level.

> [F]rom a care perspective, the morality of rights may appear callous, un-
> caringly destructive of community.[29]

"Traditional" (male) studies of moral development have set the "male"
morality of rights (on which the present legal system is based) as the standard against which the female is measured and found lacking.

The concept of "the individual" is, however, a regulatory fiction that
pervades our lives in the modern and ultramodern West. In U.S. history,
the individual is interchangeable with "the citizen": male, propertied,
heterosexually married, possessing a solitary self, a male ego with solid
boundaries, and a fixed identity.[30] The individual is necessarily dependent
on the hidden material and psychic labor of Others—women, servants,
animals, and "his" land—even as he endeavors to make his dependency
invisible.

Feminists, in debates that linger on in legal scholarship, analyzed the
opposition between care and rights. These questions have important implications for inseminating lesbians. Yet the dichotomy between care and
rights is not always as absolute as it seems, particularly for members of
disenfranchised groups who have been denied the authority and individual integrity (including the ability to participate in contracts) implied by
rights discourse. Legal scholar Patricia Williams has written powerfully
of the importance of not throwing the baby out with the bath water in
our efforts to deprivilege rights discourse. Many people are still fighting
for their rights, Williams points out, and must gain them before their importance can be reduced.[31]

Bearing in mind these limitations, feminist legal scholars have excoriated the valorization of rights discourse for all the right reasons.[32] Lesbian legal scholar Kelley Testy accurately characterizes feminist critiques of contract as "sparse but acute."

> Consistent with the central task of feminist legal theory, which is to expose male norms imbedded in the law as universal and immutable, feminist writers have criticized contract's emphasis on the bargain model of exchange. Finding the bargain model suspect because it presupposes norms of equality (of bargaining power) and freedom (to choose whether to contract), both of which have been denied to women, feminist writers have critiqued contract as a perpetuator of oppression. Contract's role in fueling a market-based economy has rendered it suspect in feminists' eyes as well, garnering it criticism for encouraging unadulterated self-interest and commodification.[33]

Finding that contract has been painted as a fixed and monolithic evil, without allowing for the complexity with which it operates in women's lives, lesbian legal scholars have begun what Testy calls "an unlikely resurrection."

> Lesbian legal theory is resurrecting contract by advocating that lesbians should seek to use contract rather than be used by it. Lesbian legal theory does this not by ignoring or obscuring aspects of contract that are problematic for feminism, but by confronting ambivalence. That is, lesbian legal theory recognizes that contract has the potential both to empower women and to oppress them.[34]

I too do not find it useful to pose a simple opposition between commodified exchange and the universe of non-commodified alternatives. Such an opposition too powerfully privileges the first term, and falls too readily into a rigid dichotomy that leaves little room for change. I also do not accept the dichotomy between care and rights. We need both.

The contract model deprivileges biological motherhood (and fatherhood), by giving all parties involved in the creation of the family equal standing in the contract (regardless of their biological involvement or gender). This arrangement could protect intentional lesbian families from both potential intrusion by the sperm donor and from the lesbian co-mother being deemed a "legal stranger" to her child(ren).

The term "stranger" was common in turn-of-the-century court decisions removing children from the care of relatives and community members and returning them to their "natural" parents.[35] It grows out of what has been called the "Adam and Eve" definition of the family, in which each family can have only one male father, one female mother, and their children. In this model, any adult who is not one of those two heteronormative parents is considered a third party and he or she has no automatic legal standing toward any children. Sometimes, in cases of a nonbiological lesbian mom seeking visitation or joint custody of children she has helped raise, the court will actually say in rejecting the claim that she cannot bring a case because she is a "legal stranger" to the child. The chill of the term, so contrary to the actual relationship between non-biological mother and child, has been frequently cited by those who would create a more inclusive definition of family.

The contractual approach might enable many lesbians to inseminate with the semen of a known donor, secure in the knowledge that he lacks the legal right to make a paternity claim. This approach has been criticized for excessive adherence to, and faith in, both contract and the legal system. Enforcing reproductive contracts, it is argued, rather than humanizing and expanding the freedom of lesbians to form families, would remove the legal protections that are still in place for mothers.[36] By legally allowing fathers to sign away their parental responsibilities, the law would strip mothers of even the nominal legal right to child support payments.[37] While its gender-neutrality is utopian, it does deprivilege the biological mother. For this reason, "contractual kinship" is both less than ideal for lesbian mother families and more likely to be realized.[38]

Redefining "Parents"

Both the "functional family" and the "contractual kinship" approach expand the definition of "parent" so that it is no longer a status comprised of one and only one male father and one and only one female mother. Approaches that seek to retain the special legal status of parents but expand who can fill that role have, understandably, been influential in lesbian family discourse.

In her 1984 article, "Rethinking Parenthood as an Exclusive Status: The Need for Legal Alternatives When the Promise of the Nuclear Family Has Failed," legal scholar Katherine Bartlett presents voluminous evidence that the exclusivity of parental status under current law is inexcusably restrictive and demonstrably harms children and other members of nonnuclear families. While Bartlett's scope is not limited to intentional lesbian families, their concerns are generously addressed. Instead of current legal definitions of parenthood, she advocates a system in which the minimum number of parents a child may have is one, thus protecting unmarried mothers from the juridical imperative to "find the child a father." There is no upper limit on the number of parents a child may have, or their genders.

Legal scholar Nancy Polikoff proposes a variation on the theme of redefining parenthood. She advocates retaining but expanding the privileged category of "parent" as above, but at the discretion of the child's biological parents. "This Child Does Have Two Mothers: Redefining Parenthood to Meet the Needs of Children in Lesbian-Mother and Other Nontraditional Families" is an encyclopedic review of case law pertaining to lesbian-mother families. In it, Polikoff promotes what she calls "equitable parenthood."[39]

In equitable parenthood, the conventional, privileged status of parents is retained, but with a Bartlett-like twist: Children are not limited to two parents, and a child's parent(s) may be of any gender. In this way, Polikoff aims to legalize lesbian as well as single-mother parenthood (which are of course overlapping categories), since the ideology of each child having two parents, one male and one female, is detrimental to children and parents in such families.

Polikoff differs from some advocates of a more voluntaristic "family registration" approach, in that she seeks to retain the special rights and status of parents in relation to their children. To this end, she proposes that under "equitable parenthood," a nonbiological parent may only gain parental status if two conditions are met. They must (1) act as a parent to the child, and (2) operate in a context where the existing parent intends that they develop a parental relationship with the child. This provision guards against what Polikoff sees as the dangerous flexibility of some "functional family" arguments, which might allow a nanny or temporary caretaker to go to court for parental standing.

In a later article, Polikoff elaborates on the anti-patriarchal effect of legally protecting families without fathers. She opens with a radically common sense statement:

> I start . . . with the premise that it is no tragedy, either on a national scale or in an individual family, for children to be raised without fathers. Children raised without love and guidance, without shelter, nutrition, and health care, without meaningful education, without physical safety in their homes and on their streets—that is tragic.[40]

After discussing the nearly impenetrable legal barriers to a woman raising children in a family without a legal father, she makes the equally striking statement:

> Statutory and doctrinal impediments to legal validation of families without fathers constitute more than a rejection of private family ordering. [A]s long as [the state] demands that every child have a legal father, [it] furthers rhetoric that a father belongs at the head of every household as the ultimate authority figure. Professor Martha Fineman observes that "the success of single mothers would be a blow to traditional masculinity." Legal validation of single mothers would be an even greater blow.

Polikoff argues that legal decisions that protect autonomous-mother families are important not only for those families—they "do more than legitimate families without fathers." These decisions present an important challenge.

> By validating such families, the decisions implicitly demand that society look elsewhere for a solution to the real problems facing today's children.[41]

The impact of such legal changes, both on individual families and family members, and on the broader cultural fabric, should not be under estimated. Redefining families is a crucial step in protecting and legitimating the families lesbians create with the help of AI.

Abolishing Marriage as a Legal Category

Legal scholar Martha Fineman presents an exceptionally complete revisioning of the family in her 1995 book, *The Neutered Mother, the Sexual Family, and Other Twentieth Century Tragedies*. Like a number of other feminist legal scholars, Fineman seeks to eliminate marriage as a legal category.[42] All adult relationships would be "private" and unregulated. What differentiates her from these other scholars is that in place of marriage, she proposes the mother-child relationship as the new core unit of the family, to be recognized, protected, and privileged by law.

Fineman rejects the "horizontal," sexual tie of husband and wife as the central unit in family formation, which, she argues, reduces children to pawns in their parents' relationships. Instead, she champions the "vertical" intimacy between mother-child as emblematic of the intimacy between caretaker and dependent, which should be the base-model for family formation. Tort, contract, and property laws would guide relationships among adults, including domestic partners, who would still have the option of being married as a religious, community, or personal ritual. With the mother-child relationship as the norm, lesbian and other unmarried mothers would no longer be stigmatized as deviant. Further, by privileging relationships that involve taking care of dependents, the "vertical family" model makes a strong statement about the value of care in society.

In essence, Fineman takes the arguments of Polikoff and the other "functional family" advocates a step farther. Where Polikoff wants the biological parents to decide whether there will be any additional parents for their child, and if so, who, Fineman wants only "Mothers" (whom she defines as nurturant caretakers of any gender) to have legal parental status. If Minow and Harlow want to expand options for who can be in legally recognized families, Fineman wants to eliminate these "sexual" families from the purview of the law. If some lesbian activists want to abolish marriage as a fundamentally flawed institution, Fineman wants to abolish not only marriage but also any parenthood other than that of nurturant mothers. She is among the most radical of current feminist family law scholars.

Why, Fineman asks, should the intimate partners of mothers (whether they are biological genitors or not) be allowed or expected to co-parent, when the sexual relationship (between men and women, and in same-sex couples) is the least stable and permanent of all intimate bonds? Why not instead institutionalize protection for the intimate relationships most in need of and deserving of it, that is, mother-child? This is the unit that must be nurtured and supported in order to reproduce the population, and this is the unit in which both "inevitable dependencies" (i.e., of children) and "secondary dependencies" (i.e., of mothers involved in taking care of them) inhere. Adding fathers, or same-sex partners who occupy a family role similar to that of fathers, into the official family unit is, according to Fineman, asking for trouble. Rather, let us empower mothers, protect and support their relationships with their children and community.

If mothers want to have mates, life partners, or lovers of any gender, those people can have access to relationships with the children if the mother judges it in her child's best interest. One strength of this approach stems from its recognition of the utter lack of equivalence between mothers and fathers. This lack of equivalence is inseparable from the fact that women and men are not equal in society, no matter how much we would like them to be. These differences in power cannot be conveniently classified as either "biological" or "socially constructed." I have come to believe that something being "socially constructed" simply means it is probably less amenable to change than if it were strictly "biological," in which case it might be changed through biomedical intervention. As legal scholar Catherine MacKinnon writes,

> The intractability of maleness as a form of dominance suggests that social constructs, although they flow from human agency, can be less plastic than nature has proven to be. If experience trying to do so is any guide, it may be easier to change biology than society.[43]

Regardless of how we explain their origins, inequalities between motherhood and fatherhood exist, along with important differences within those categories. Women make an infinitely greater and more sacrificial contribution to procreation than do men. This imbalance continues into the care and nurture of babies, children, and dependent adults. Because of these and many other real differences, it is not useful to act as if men and women, mothers and fathers, are "equal" in medicine, families, or the law.

Medically, donating semen is not the same as donating ova. Women have a limited number of eggs (although far more than they could use in a lifetime), whereas men typically produce sperm in astronomical numbers— three to five million per ejaculation. Comparing semen donation with egg donation is something like comparing producing a urine sample to having one's wisdom teeth removed. Only therein lies the problem—there is no valid comparison.

When people try to level motherhood and fatherhood medically, we find ourselves in the realm of the ridiculous homology, where gender-neutral language reduces eggs and sperm to equivalent "gametes" that are legally leveled and governed by the same standards. In these cases, the law cannot recognize the difference between a sperm donor and a mother, and will thus grant equal parental standing to both.

What the male models of parenthood take for granted is that the male body is the standard, the yardstick by which everyone else is measured. Just as the law once found women inferior due to their "difference" from men, now the law measures women by the "same" standards as men and finds them lacking. Clearly, both essentialist and social constructionist discourses can be used against the rights of lesbians, women, and mothers.

Men's and women's bodies have much in common and much that is different. Whether similarities or differences are emphasized is a political matter and subject to change. For instance, sexologists in the 1960s and 1970s who "proved" the similarities between male and female sexual responses challenged the long-standing scientific emphasis on the differences between male and female physiology.[44] Creating homologies between men's and women's bodies may be politically useful for lesbians in some instances. In the arena of procreation and child rearing, such leveling can be catastrophic.

While the desire to locate power differentials in biology is historically linked to sexist, racist, and eugenicist ideology, the denial of mothers' stronger social bonds to children has also been used against women. Pretending there is such a thing as gender-neutral "parenting" has been disastrous for women. In large part this is because biological and social mothering is one of the only areas where women are at an "advantage" to men in relation to their children since women can have babies and men (as of yet) cannot. Nurturant fatherhood is more prevalent today than a generation ago.[45] Still, mothers and other women provide the vast majority of nurturing to children (as well as to other family members).[46] Much as we may struggle to change the gendered division of labor in child rearing, denial of the facts has proved costly for women. A prime example of catastrophic legal denial of mothers' "difference" is the U.S. abolition, in the 1970s, of maternal custody preferences at divorce. The shift from the presumption of maternal custody to the doctrine of "the best interests of the child" was fought for and hailed by feminists in the 1970s. The gender-neutral language that replaced the privileging of mothers was seen as a feminist victory against the sexist cultural assumptions that women were necessarily maternal, and that men could not be nurturing caretakers. Unfortunately, such gender-blind legal language made for profoundly sexist law.

When mothers had to compete with fathers to prove that they were better parents, the fathers almost always came out ahead because fathers generally had more money (and were thus seen as being "better able to provide for the child") and because fathers could generally present themselves more sympathetically to male judges. They could also marry new "mothers" for the children. The threat of a traumatic custody battle now hangs like a pall over mothers, who need to be concerned that, if the parents split up for whatever reason, the father will probably win custody if he wants it.

It is a widespread myth that mothers are given preference in custody battles. In fact, men rarely sue for custody. When they do, they win it about two-thirds of the time. Massachusetts' fathers are more than three times more likely than mothers to win custody cases.[47] Mothers only get custody of children in such a majority of divorces because fathers generally do not seek it.[48] Still, fathers can now "play the custody card" to negotiate favorable conditions (low or no child support or alimony) in a divorce settlement, which contributes to the feminization of poverty, the disadvantaging of mothers in the legal system, and the disempowerment of women. Abusive fathers use custody suits and the threat of custody suits to abuse mothers further and keep them trapped in abusive relationships.

For these and many other reasons, motherhood and fatherhood are not the same, even though there is a spectrum of each, with significant overlaps. Therefore, the way to give women more power than they have now (perhaps even someday approaching "equality" with men) is not to deny the realities of patriarchy, such as male economic and legal power, but to fight for more power for women. Since motherhood is a central arena in which women are disadvantaged, it is a crucial arena for feminist struggle.

Central to Fineman's argument is the awareness that society fails to acknowledge the inevitable dependencies that are inherent in the life cycle.

This denial is part of an American ethos that valorizes and rewards "capitalistic individualism, independence, self-sufficiency, and autonomy."[49] Caretakers cannot measure up to this yardstick. Because mothers and other caretakers, overwhelmingly women, also need support to do their caretaking work, they are secondarily dependent. This "secondary dependence" leaves mothers with needs that require special legal and social consideration. Expecting mothers to behave as self-sufficient breadwinners, Fineman points out, has the dual effect of diverting attention from our collective social responsibility for mothers and children and letting the state off the hook.

As legal scholar M.M. Slaughter points out, "The refusal to recognize that dependents cannot stand alone comes from a restricted vision of human relationships and results in a denial of the value of caring for others."[50] This devaluation of the work of care, in and out of the family, typifies a masculinist ethos that has pervasive, destructive effects on the social fabric.[51] The bulk of the damage is wrought on the most clearly dependent: children, the elderly, the seriously ill or disabled, and their caretakers. As Fineman and others suggest, no amount of "help" by a partner can make up for the societal devaluing of caring work. Until society values and supports mothers and those who need mothering, regardless of mothers' sexual and legal attachments to men, the family will remain profoundly gendered, and the impoverishment of mothers and children will continue.

Advocating the primacy of motherhood in child rearing has powerful ramifications for lesbian and feminist empowerment. Alternative insemination among lesbians is one small area where women are struggling for power, self-determination, and autonomy from men. Lesbians who inseminate, and their families, buck the heteropatriarchal imperative in several regards. They live as lesbians, rejecting compulsory heterosexuality. They have children without men, rejecting the imperative that every child must have a father. And they reject the totalizing phallic imaginary, which Monique Wittig has called "The Straight Mind," by changing the terms on which their lives will be lived. Wittig first identifies the oppressive discourses.

> The discourses which particularly oppress all of us, lesbians, women, and homosexual men, are those discourses which take for granted that

what founds society, any society, is heterosexuality. These discourses speak about us and claim to say the truth in an apolitical field . . . as if, in what concerns us, politically insignificant signs could exist.[52]

Wittig describes the damage these discourses do as being both in a realm of ideas and very real:

> These discourses of heterosexuality oppress us in the sense that they prevent us from speaking unless we speak in their terms. These discourses deny us every possibility of creating our own categories. But their most ferocious action is the unrelenting tyranny that they exert upon our physical and mental selves.

New legal definitions of the family, according to Fineman, must center around those who are dependent on others for their care, including children, the elderly and the ill, as well as on their caretakers (currently almost always women) who need support in order to do the work of caretaking. Toward this end, we are all served by flexibility in adult (horizontal) relationships and continuity in dependent (vertical) relationships. In the midst of all these shifting familial contours, there is a pressing need for responsibility amidst the confusion as well as pleasure in constructing new boundaries.[53]

Fineman's vision has been criticized for its focus on women's maternity at the expense of their sexuality. For instance, Slaughter, while finding Fineman's critique of the nuclear family "utterly convincing," takes issue with the prospect of deprivileging sexuality within the family:

> Because of its focus on the mother/child relationship as the core of the family, however, Fineman's proposal may also deny and exclude feminine sexuality. It suppresses an essential element of women's public identity even though that element may be antagonistic to patriarchy and the demands of the work ethic. Rather than subordinate sexuality (as patriarchs insist) or make it private (as Fineman suggests), I argue that women must claim public recognition of, and respect for, both their maternal and sexual natures.[54]

Such a critique seems particularly salient when it comes to lesbian mothers' complex negotiation of their maternal and sexual identities. Legally deprivileging sexual relationships, however, will not necessarily lead to further marginalization of lesbians or further invisibility of lesbian eroticism and relationships. To the contrary, if adult sexual relationships were legally privatized, a massive leveling of all kinds of adult relationships would take place. Heteropatriarchal sexuality, marriage, and kinship are so extremely valorized and legally privileged, that eliminating laws that prop up heteropatriarchy would be a far-reaching move to empower intentional lesbian families and all kinds of heterogeneous families. If, in addition, maternal families were centered legally, with the valuation of caring work that that would imply, a fundamental blow would have been dealt to compulsory heterosexuality. By loosening the heteropatriarchal imperative, lesbian eroticism, far from being sacrificed, might have the social space to proliferate as never before. Moving adult relationships into the "private" realm, stripping them of both state sanction and state censure, would not abolish them. Rather it would, at least in theory, go a long way toward eliminating the social controls that now inhibit creation and maintenance of voluntary horizontal intimacies.

Many who favor deprivileging biology, including the advocates of gender-neutral contractual procreation, would surely object to Fineman's vision. However, even feminists who object to "biological essentialism" might be willing to make an exception if it means empowering mothers in child rearing and the law.

Lesbian mothers would be empowered at least as much as heterosexual mothers, though in different ways, if Fineman's objectives were enacted. Even more than through same-sex marriage, lesbians would gain instant legal parity between their relationships and heterosexual relationships, all of which would be unregulated—neither privileged nor denigrated— by the law. Lesbians, like all women, could have children, with or without others, without the fear of paternal claims from genitors. And the conditions of women's motherhood would not be contingent upon, or even necessarily linked to, their horizontal relationship status. Women, including lesbians, could find themselves in a utopia of maternal empowerment.

Criticisms of Fineman's approach are pointed. In addition to skepticism about the practicability of eliminating marriage as a legal category, critics point out that Fineman's approach is not oriented toward lesbians, and would not enhance the legal or social status of (nonbiological) co-mothers.

And the radical nature of the changes Fineman advocates makes her proposal unlikely to be realized soon.

Working for Children's Rights

Some scholars argue that the way out of the conundrums of defining the family is to shift the focus from the adults to the children, and in particular to emphasize children's rights. Children historically were considered the property of their fathers in U.S. (and much of European) common law, and they are still treated as such by many adults, including those in the judiciary. A laissez-faire ethic of children as property pervades U.S. policy toward children of all social classes. The stark absence of prenatal and child care, the widespread poverty of children, and the prevalence of physical and sexual child abuse lay bare our collective devaluation of children in the United States.[55] One could argue that the children of the wealthy are valued in U.S. society, and certainly they are much more highly valued than the children of the poor. Yet wealthy fathers share with poor fathers an abysmal record on providing court-ordered child support payments.[56]

A children's rights perspective would bring the child's "needs, values, dignity, and experiences" front and center in family law and policy considerations.[57] The needs and rights of the adult claimants would be subordinated to those of the child. The child's needs, for love, care and continuity in her important relationships, including especially the child's "network of care," would be the standard by which custody, visitation, and other family-related decisions would be made.[58] In a study of "reproductive technologics, surrogacy, adoption, and same-sex and unwed parents," political scientist Mary Lyndon Shanley concludes that a child-centered approach is necessary to a fair and just family policy that can accommodate the range of existing family forms.

> A child-centered approach to family policy requires that the law protect relationships that are fundamental to a child's sense of self and well being, including the parental status of a lesbian nonbiological mother. It is the recognition of a child's right to a permanent, nurturing relationship, more than of an adult's right to parent a child, that is the proper

grounding of the parental status of biological and nonbiological parents alike.[59]

This approach seems infinitely preferable to the typical focus on parental rights, in which the child becomes a pawn in battles between adults. Shanley points out that a child-centered approach would "ground" the claims of the nonbiological lesbian mother in the child's "need for and right to her care," not in "the entitlements of adults."[60]

A children's rights approach does not assume that children are qualified to function as adults. Children and infants are dependent on adults, and deserve protection as well as rights. A child's developmental stage must be taken into account when considering her wishes. Children's rights would put the children's perspective at the center.

In theory, the "best interest of the child" standard does the same thing. In reality, courts often will not consider the child's best interests relevant unless the parent is unfit or has abandoned the child.[61] In the "best interest" standard, the child's interests are mediated by adults who presume to speak for the child. So judges in cases involving lesbian mothers have referred to the "right" of a child to have both a mother and a father, and the "right" of a child to grow up in a "normal" (non-lesbian) family.

Some authors suggest that truly child-centered family law would minimize such excesses of judicial discretion in determining the child's best interest.[62] Instead of simply taking the child's opinions as evidence in a hearing, the child's stated wishes would be given the status of testimony and honored whenever possible. A central goal would be to "give voice" to the child and to see things from her perspective. Legal scholar Barbara Bennett Woodhouse suggests five human rights principles that can be adapted and applied to children's unique position:

> The equality principle becomes the right to equal opportunity.
> The individualism principle becomes the right to be treated as a unique individual and not as an object.
> The privacy principle honors the child's intimate relationships.
> The protection principle requires government to protect the weak from the strong.
> The empowerment principle supports the child's right to a voice in court proceedings.[63]

If such principles were enshrined in law, as part of a larger move to care for children, they could give structure to the currently amorphous "best interest of the child" standard. They would also protect lesbian families, since most judicial decisions denying the co-mother's standing, or granting parental status to the donor, violate the child's needs, rights, and wishes.

Children are currently not given the power to decide their own custody arrangements in part because of the belief that children are not mature enough to identify their own interests, and in part to protect the child from manipulation and coercion by one or both parents. These concerns point to the major divide within the children's rights movement. Simply stated, on one side is the belief that children need to be protected, and on the other is the belief that children need to be empowered.[64] Both of these tendencies are represented in the international treaties on the rights of the child (e.g., the 1989 *Convention on the Rights of the Child* [CRC]) and both are crucial parts of the international children's rights agenda.

Making the linkages between children's rights in lesbian family contests—custody disputes, second-parent adoption efforts, same-sex marriage and domestic partnership campaigns—and the movement for children's rights overall, might well be an effective tactic in specific instances. A nonbiological lesbian mother could ground her claims for a continuing relationship with her children after a breakup with the biological mother in part on Article Five of the CRC:

> States Parties [countries] shall respect the responsibilities, rights and duties of parents or, *where applicable, the members of the extended family or community as provided for by local custom,* legal guardians or other persons legally responsible for the child, to provide, in a manner consistent with the evolving capacities of the child, appropriate direction and guidance in the exercise by the child of the rights recognized in the present Convention. [Emphasis added.]

The CRC is a powerful document that enshrines the rights of every child in the world to a life of dignity and fulfillment. The United States is one of two countries in the world that have yet to ratify this convention, the other being Somalia. It has signed the convention, however, signaling its intention to ratify. Nonetheless, even when such human rights conventions are not ratified, they can do powerful work. In addition to articulating international standards, and moral suasion, the use of such documents helps to build a larger culture of human rights that benefits us all.

The Importance of Vision

Legal scholar John Vagelatos has compared Fineman to the mythical prophet Cassandra, who could speak the truth but was destined to go unheeded. Vagelatos points out that

> while change may not come in the form which Fineman advocates, its radical nature makes it difficult to be co-opted by the dominant ideology, forcing discourse outside of traditional boundaries.[65]

Even though a utopian vision of change such as Fineman's is unlikely to have immediate practical application, it still plays an important part in the process of legal and cultural change.

By providing an ideal against which to measure not only our present situation but also our strategies toward reform, visionaries provide crucial inspiration, energy, and hope for people in the trenches. All oppressed groups need to be able to envision a world where our oppression does not seem preordained as natural. There must be a visionary wing in all social movements to keep it focused and spiritually alive. It cannot be the only wing—but it is vital. Robin West articulates the importance of imagining beyond immediate crises as well as taking concrete steps to redress them. She envisions a utopian, feminist jurisprudence.

> Feminism must envision a post-patriarchal world, for without such a vision we have little direction. We must use that vision to construct our present goals, and we should, I believe, interpret our present victories against the backdrop of that vision. . ..
>
> In a utopian world . . . a perfect legal system will protect against harms sustained by all forms of life, and will recognize life-affirming values generated by all forms of being. Feminist jurisprudence must aim to bring this about and, to do so, must aim to transform the images as well as the power.[66]

While Fineman's (and others') proposals may remain mythically in the realm of discourse, they help move that discourse in the direction of justice for intentional lesbian families. Judging by the volume of serious responses to Fineman and Polikoff's work, such scholars are not necessarily doomed to share Cassandra's fate.

The Lesbian Mother Closet

It is a tragedy that despite all the aforementioned possibilities, the closet may still be the most prevalent strategy that intentional lesbian mothers (and all lesbian and gay parents) use to try to safeguard their families. Sometimes the closet is the most effective approach given the heterosexist circumstances in which most lesbians raise children. Being discreet, lying when necessary, living a double life, and avoiding controversy that might draw attention to one's lesbianism are survival strategies to which most lesbian mothers are forced to resort. While the psychic violence of the closet, and the material and social violence that sustain it, are well known among lesbians and gay men, scholars are only beginning to document the devastation wrought on children who must grow up in the terror, hiding, and self-surveillance of the family closet. Living in fear that a slip of the tongue may result in the destruction of one's livelihood, housing, physical safety, community, and/or family are burdensome enough for an adult. How much more unbearable for the child who risks inadvertently raining ruin on her mother's life.[67]

The solution to the ills of the closet is not just "coming out" for the individual lesbian mother, a decision that may be eminently unsafe for her family. Rather, the solution lies in changing the heterosexism that pervades our psychosocial fabric and manifests as personal, interpersonal, cultural, and institutional homophobia.[68]

The Lesbian-Normative Universe

Countless lesbians are creating and sustaining cultures that promote lesbian family well-being. Theirs is a strategy of staying alive in a culture that despises them. Countless lesbians work and live in ways that sustain a lesbian *"nomos"*—a "normative universe"—of which lesbian AI is a part. As legal scholar Thomas Ross explains, "The *nomos* is composed only in part of the rules and institutions we commonly identify as our legal structure. Our *nomos* is also composed of the stories we tell." Ross elaborates the idea of a "feminist *nomos*" in *Just Stories: How the Law Embodies Racism and Bias.* Ross defines *nomos* as "a normative universe that is as much a part of our existence as the physical world we inhabit within which we constantly create and maintain a world of right and wrong, of lawful and unlawful, of valid and void."[69]

The idea of a lesbian-normative universe is useful for theorizing lesbian AI. For me, a lesbian-normative universe is not a mere mirror image of heteronormativity, only this time with lesbianism being equated with humanity. Rather, a lesbian-normative universe is cosmically compatible with all kinds of lesbian-friendly sexual and kinship constellations. Most importantly, a lesbian-normative universe puts lesbians at the center, rather than trying to fit them into existing heteropatriarchal norms.

In the face of institutional disempowerment, lesbians have created alternative discourses and institutions to support their access to insemination and motherhood. This lesbian culture-building lays bare the sexism, heterosexism, and social-constructedness of the seemingly value-neutral medical uses of AI. Lesbians have changed AI, and in the process have problematized some of the smooth machinery of patriarchal discourses. Creating and raising families outside of patriarchal paradigms, inseminating lesbians and their families are forced to invent alternative theories to justify and bolster their family practices. These lived alternatives to nuclear family, compulsory heterosexuality, the naturalization of kinship, and heteronormative ideology have given rise to a growing body of "street theory."[70] This theory stands in marked contrast to the legal theory embedded in social institutions, with which inseminating lesbians must contend. These emergent paradigms are circulated in a lesbian culture that builds institutions as well as discourses.

Lesbian narratives about AI and motherhood, for instance, support a normative universe in which lesbians and their families get to survive. Such discourses, which are lesbian-positive, and which are not "sustained by the threat of our unnatural horror," make all the difference. The continual sustaining of a "normative" lesbian community in which lesbians and their families may thrive, are just as crucial as the struggles with the legal and medical establishments discussed throughout this book. The stories, legal and otherwise, of intentional lesbian families, give lie to the unarticulated anti-lesbian stories that underlie, and are codified in, the state's law.[71]

To the extent that lesbian mothers' legal arguments do this, they participate in the creation of lesbian normative universe that serves to bolster lesbians.[72] Thus the activities of pro-lesbian activists, in and out of the legal arena, contribute to that aspect of the law that is redemptive, rather than to the dominant aspect, which is not.

Such a normative universe must necessarily include both non-heteropatriarchal kinship and non-heteropatriarchal economics. Lesbian AI contributes substantially to this universe by engaging in both alternative kinship and alternative forms of trade.

As the whole concept of the *nomos* suggests, it is not only those who are engaging in lesbian AI who contribute to that normative universe. Those who contribute to the culture, legal status, medical recognition, and family integrity of inseminating lesbians also play a crucial role, as do those whose writing, speaking, and envisioning help legitimate them. Such supporting activities are not just about that *nomos* but are part of it. It is my strong hope that this book will be a useful part of that process, which is about the survival and well-being of real people in real families.

Intentional Lesbian Family Futures

We might begin to imagine possible (utopian) scenarios if we project out the impact of lesbian AI and its *nomos* into the future. In such a future, the nuclear family is demoted to one among many family forms in which people may choose to live and raise children. As a culture, we shift from a formal-legal-patriarchal to a "dependency" model of procreation. In such a system, embryos, fetuses, babies, and children are understood to be primarily bonded with, to "belong to," the adults who take care of them—certainly until birth, and usually long after, these are mothers. Genetics are of decidedly secondary relevance, and vertical intimacies are valued and protected. Until such time as a genitor establishes a social relationship with his child or children, he has the status of "sperm donor."[73] This scenario fosters creative and flexible forms of kinship and family networks.

In this world, men relate to and care for children not as the patriarchal owner-fathers of feudal times, not as the rigidly gendered breadwinners of the 1950s, and not as the alienated strangers of the 1970s, 1980s, and 1990s. In this scenario, men relate to others, including children, not as property or heirs or namesakes or reflections of their masculinity or social status. In this scenario, men, like women, relate to children as flesh and blood human beings, because they too have human needs for kinship, bonding, enduring intimacies, and love.

This is the kind of system that is already incipient in the current self-insemination movement (along with its opposing trend of atomized consumerism). The practice of lesbian AI is both discursively supported by and materially enacts such woman- and mother-centered discourses, ethics, and *nomos* about the roles of women, men, and babies.

Despite the problems involved with AI, it remains an important liberatory technology for lesbians and other women, and expands the boundaries of the family in ways that, overall, increase our social freedom. Lesbian AI creates new spaces of socially responsible electivity for the simple reason that it is mother-centered, and based on choice independent of social mandate. The more women exercise their freedom to make independent choices about kinship and sexuality, the more freedom it creates for others. When lesbian families are living openly on a block, and their children are in the neighborhood school, all the children grow up with an increased sense of possibilities for their lives. These options are important for all women, lesbian or not, if we believe that women are not flowerpots made for growing men's seed.[74]

As a postmodern social form, lesbian AI takes full advantage of medical technology, of the loosening discursive grip of the nuclear family as hegemonic referent, and of the commodified lifestyle choice of childbearing and -rearing. Yet it also practices pro-kinship values, as it constitutes a radical stand for intimacy and embodied kinship, without calling for a "return" to an idealized, naturalized, and patriarchal family. Crucially, every AI child is a wanted child, or at least a pursued one.

At the same time, intentional lesbian families reject the reactionary "family values" of those who long with nostalgia for an innocence that never existed for women who have historically been the currency of exchange in "natural" arrangements among men. Such nostalgia for a romantically imagined state of natural harmony is untenable for lesbians who have long been considered unnatural. Intentional lesbian families, by definition, are inclined to reject the naturalization of any form of patriarchal kinship arrangements. Instead, they participate in, and in different degrees strive for, the dismantling of heteropatriarchy.

Motherhood, as the magical sign of womanhood, has been historically constrained within the patriarchal family if it was to be considered "legitimate." "I am a mother because I am married because I am heterosexual because I am a woman because I am a mother." Lesbian inseminators break this tautological chain. Within a lesbian family context, these naturalized identities are reversed and displaced. With AI, lesbians reject these values, and claim the prerogatives of intentional motherhood. Alternative insemination becomes a form of "immasculate conception": the closest thing we humans have to parthenogenesis.[75]

Inseminating lesbians benefit from at least some men's alienation from their semen, and from the larger male flight from familial intimacies. But lesbian AI is not primarily about the flight from intimacy. Rather, it transmutes social conditions of alienation to create mother(s)- and-child-centered families.

Lesbian AI can be seen as helping to pave the way for the kind of mother-centered kinship structure that Fineman envisions, in which caring is socially valued both inside and outside the home, and in which men and other women are invited to participate based on the mother's wishes. This utopia involves a different foundation for the social order than those of capitalism and patriarchy—one that is based on care, intimacy, social responsibility, and interdependence. This scenario is based on moving toward a world beyond the sex/gender binary, where an exuberance of sexes, genders, and sexualities can flourish. A world beyond patriarchy. A world that I would not mind living in.

Appendix A

Methodology, Sources, and Citations

My research is multidisciplinary, transdisciplinary, and sometimes even counterdisciplinary. I use a combination of quantitative and qualitative methodologies, with a strong preference toward the latter. I consider my work to be both humanistic and interpretive. A sociologist by trade, I also do not shy away from political science or legal scholarship methodologies when appropriate. I draw from a wide range of sources, which I read against each other using analytic frames drawn from feminist theory, queer theory, and cultural and literary studies, as well as sociology.[1] Some readers may be accustomed to a more linear approach to scholarly writing, in which there is one "primary" point toward which all of the "lesser" points are directed, so that all chapters lead to a single logical conclusion. Such readers may find this book somewhat different. Like its subject, it is characterized by a multiplicity of points, no two alike, each one connected to the others by webs of transferential meaning, as in acupuncture. Acupuncture, as practiced in North America, is an ancient Chinese system of diagnosis and healing. Its view of the body is complex, subtle, and holistic. The body is seen as a system of energy affected by diet, feelings, and environment, among other factors. Its understanding of the body is organized around such concepts as yin and yang, the internal organs, and the five elements of fire, wind, wood, earth, and water, all of which must be in dynamic balance.

In Chinese acupuncture, the body contains energy pathways ("meridians") associated with the organs, which can be either blocked or flooded. The energy flowing through them can be too fast or too slow, too hot or too cold, or out of balance with other meridians/organs. Each meridian can be drawn as a line on the human body. The kidney meridian, for example, runs along the arch of one's foot, up the webbing below the inner ankle, and around to the top of the front lateral calf muscle. Each meridian has "points" on which energy in the organs can be adjusted with needles, heat, or manual stimulation. These points are each meaningful, and in complex relationship with each other.

Two patients presenting with identical symptoms may be diagnosed, and thus treated, very differently. So my insomnia might be caused by "deficient kidney chi" (energy), and yours could be caused by "blood heat." The Western doctor, perceiving the same symptom, might give us the same sleeping pill. (The doctor might also ignore our concerns or offer us pills from pharmaceutical marketers.) The acupuncturist might place slim needles below my navel. She might place thicker needles above your inner knee. The acupuncturist looks at the whole patient, including body, mind, and environment. The Western physician is trained to overlook the whole patient and focus instead on the symptoms and treatment of illness.

What is the primary acupuncture point? That question misses the point. The points are part of a system (of lines that flow), and only make sense in relation to each other. One set of points is highlighted at a certain time, for a certain patient. Another set of points is highlighted at another time.

In this book, I map out my discussion of lesbian AI somewhat like the acupuncturist's points on the body. I want to understand the whole body of lesbian AI. I map this body from several angles, and in several of its elements. I am asking a general question: What is going on here? I have a general argument: This matters.

Inseminating lesbians and their families are affected by the situation of women, of mothers, of those who inseminate, of "queers," of the many other demographic groups into which they fall. I discuss several of the major meridians in the body of lesbian AI, as well as some of the more relevant points that comprise them. Law, medicine, and the family are major organs, with intersecting meridians. Some of the most powerful points are where these lines intersect, and I give them special attention.

My methodology has a strong affinity with "socioacupuncture." "Socioacupuncture" is a term coined by author and Native American Studies scholar Gerald Vizenor, and presented in his essay "Socioacupuncture: Mythic Reversals and the Striptease in Four Acts." In this complex, multi-layered, and brilliant work, Vizenor connects socioacupuncture with what he calls a "liberatory tribal striptease." In this striptease, the dancer ritually undoes the violent freezing of Native American creativity, culture, and humanity that is typified in white men's fetishized photographs that claim to portray "authentic" Native Americans. In the process, the dancer playfully, "deliciously" reclaims power to disrupt some of the genocidal immobility that Euro-American colonialism has imposed. Vizenor writes,

> The striptease is the prime form of socioacupuncture, a therapeutic tease and technique, which is accomplished through tribal trickeries and mythic satire, eternal contradictions that release the ritual terror in captured images.[2]

The term socioacupuncture resonates with me on a number of levels. It is a "delicious" form of anti-imperialist praxis. It is a simultaneously powerful and humorous analytic framework. It is an acknowledgment of the bodies in question and a desire for healing. It is a lens/method that privileges flows of energy more than biomedicalistic dissections, both corporeal and analytical. I also find socioacupuncture a useful method with which to approach the analysis of discourses. Discourses, again, are not merely conversation, but the place where power and knowledge unite, where domination and resistance to domination battle in a variety of institutional and "private" settings. Discourses are flexible, fluid even, and can be deployed, with various degrees of intentionality, toward various goals at different times or places. As Foucault notes,

> Just as the network of power relations ends by forming a dense web that passes through apparatuses and institutions, without being exactly localized in them, so too the swarm of points of resistance traverses social stratifications and individual unities.[3]

These networks, swarms, webs, and non-localized flows of power and resistance seem particularly subject to the (metaphorical) analyses and interventions of socioacupuncture. Socioacupuncture is an alternative to positivism, a "pagan" epistemology if you will.[4] Pagan epistemologies "are a descent out of what is hegemonically taken for granted, that creates mythic openings for alternative futures."[5] Socioacupuncture calls into question how we know what we know, challenging the "common sense" of the status quo.

Pagan epistemologies assert the reality of social flux against the dominance of the isolated individual who is supported by phallic ideologies. They imply connection, continuity, compassionate awareness of our existence in the food chain, and the recognition of the intrinsic value (as opposed to the exchange value or use value) of beings. Pagan epistemologies reject the zero-sum game of taxonomizing bodies, the body/mind split, and the body that is rigidly gendered, racialized, and organized by national and sexual legal categories. They assert a more generous exchange of boundaries as well as the utter interdependency of bodies for survival. In good sociological tradition, pagan epistemologies attend to the invisible as well as the visible, and labor to sustain a compassionate sense of irony (making the mundane strange and the strange mundane) about our fragile and complex common conditions.

My approach, like the practices and relations of lesbian AI, is ultramodern. Socioacupuncture is inventive, dissenting, conventional, utopian, partial, and ambivalent. Take as an example the vexing problem of trying to establish the size of the "lesbian baby boom" in general, and the number of lesbians engaging in AI in particular. How many lesbians inseminate each year? How many lesbians have inseminated overall? How many children have been born whom lesbians conceived via AI?[6]

To try to answer these questions I did the following:

- Read the major peer-reviewed studies of lesbians, lesbian families, and lesbian insemination practices.
- Found social science, legal, medical, and popular articles specifically on the topic of lesbian AI and noted their estimates, as well as the sources given for the estimates (if available).
- Searched the social science literature (sociology, psychology, political science) to see what figures are standard when estimating the number of lesbians in the United States and what sources are cited for them.
- Searched the medical literature to find out what research has been done on AI in

the United States and abroad, and noted their figures as to how many inseminations are performed each year.

- Referred to the official statistics cited by authorities such as infertility societies in the United States and abroad, tissue bank societies, and government-sponsored research in the United States and abroad.
- Obtained estimates from sperm banks of both the number of inseminations they perform each year (when available) and estimates as to how many of their clients are lesbians and/or unmarried.
- Searched the major lesbian and LGBT organizations' fact sheets and websites to see their numbers for both lesbians and lesbian AI. I noted their sources (if available).
- Tried to ascertain how the various sources were defining "lesbian" and how reliable those definitions were.
- Followed up on sources cited, got a picture of the claims, stakes, and other issues involved in tracking these numbers.
- Stayed receptive to serendipitous sources of information and ways of looking at and getting at the problem.
- Finally, made my best guesses based on the evidence I could find, while acknowledging that I could still be off target.

My sources include the following:

Lexis/Nexis (supplemented by help from legal librarians at Suffolk University and Harvard University law schools) for information and analysis about all things legal;

Medical journals, for medical research and analysis of lesbian insemination and lesbians;

Social science scholarship—drawn from disciplines including sociology, anthropology, political science, and psychology, as well as interdisciplinary fields such as women's studies and queer theory—for data and analysis about lesbian insemination and family practices;

National and international lesbian, feminist, and LGBT organizations for summaries and analysis of relevant issues, policies, laws, and trends;

Popular lesbian, feminist, and LGBT media for keeping abreast of these perspectives on trends and issues;

Mainstream print media for keeping abreast of mainstream perspectives on the issues;

Sperm bank literature, including donor profiles, fee schedules, and fact sheets;

U.S. and international medical societies, especially fertility societies, including protocols and position papers, conference proceedings, and other publications for the official medical perspective on insemination and other forms of commercial and contractual reproduction, and views about lesbians using them;

Websites related to all of the above;

Informal interviews, conversations, and first-hand knowledge.

The above constitute socioacupuncture in several ways. I tried to read each number as part of a larger discourse that has stakes in the facts presented. I read the divergent counts as symptomatic of larger disputes among the parties reporting them, disputes about bigger issues than the number of lesbians inseminating, disputes that resound in the larger body politic. I looked at my efforts to find the range of views on the scope of lesbian AI as not only a straightforward quest for the truth, but also as a marker for larger issues. It was a non-linear process. Finally, I undertook this process in part out of a desire for healing.

Because my sources are so varied, a word about my citation practices may be helpful. I adhere to normal academic citation practices whenever possible. When several sources provide the same information, I try to cite the originator. However, when information is factual (e.g., which countries have anti-lesbian laws), I try to cite a source that is easy for the reader to access. If I am aware that a friend or colleague gave me an idea, I will acknowledge it. When referring to legal cases and other matters of public record, I cite the original documents when possible, in addition to whichever law journal or other secondary sources I may use.

Appendix B

Definitions

One of my goals in this book is to arrive at language that is both empowering and faithful to those it represents. Who has, or ought to have, the power to define AI and the families affected by it remains contested. By now it is axiomatic that we can never assume a representation is neutral or objective. Rather, all representations issue from people who occupy specific standpoints and articulate interests and values. In the arena of procreative technologies, the practices are so new that the words used to describe them effectively determine their perception and reception by society at large. As always, the accounts themselves are sociological phenomena.[1] This section includes definitions of key terms I use throughout the book.

Lesbian

Lesbians have been arguing about what a lesbian *really* is for many years. If you open a lesbian, feminist, or LGBT publication today, popular or academic, you are likely to find some effort to define what a lesbian is, was, or should be. The terms of the debates change over time, but the question remains open.

Some of the debates hinge on the question of electivity. Can (or should) every woman become a lesbian? Or is lesbianism an inborn, or early-childhood-fixed sexual orientation that people have no control over? Are there "primary" lesbians who *only* want to be with women and "secondary" lesbians who *could* be with men but choose lesbianism for other reasons (e.g., egalitarian relationships, reduced risks of sexually transmitted infections, freedom from contraception), and for whom lesbian sexuality is a less important consideration?

Another discussion centers on the gendered nature of lesbian existence. Are lesbians more woman-identified than other women, since they live a woman-centered life without male partners? Or, on the contrary, are lesbians gender-benders, transgressing the boundaries between woman and man?

Yet another dispute hinges on the defining characteristics of lesbians. Is a lesbian someone who is sexual with other women? Can you still be a lesbian if you are sexual with men, or if you have never (yet) been sexual with women? Is desire a sufficient qualifier— is a lesbian someone who *wants* to have sexual relationships with other women? Or, to use the U.S. military's terms, is lesbianism a *status* rather than a form of *conduct?* In other words, is stating that you are a lesbian enough to qualify you as one, regardless of what you *do* about it? Conversely, is a woman who has sexual relationships only with women, but who denies that she is a lesbian, still a lesbian? Are lesbians the vanguard of the feminist movement, and heterosexuals and bisexuals less politically committed to feminism? Or are lesbians just women who are sexually attracted to other women, plain and simple? Or rather is lesbian existence a spiritual condition, defined by a unique, magical, and possibly two-spirited soul?

Should we view lesbian existence as a continuum, with all women having some amount of bonding with other women, and therefore existing somewhere on the continuum? Are all people bisexual to some extent? If so, is it divisive to use the category "lesbian" at all? Would it be better to stop separating people into such rigid categories and just focus on being human, without labels? Is the term "lesbian" a kind of regulatory fiction, a category of social control? After all, didn't voyeuristic and misogynist scientists invent the categories of "homosexual" and "heterosexual"? Should we call ourselves "gay" or "queer" instead of "lesbian," in order to identify ourselves with a larger, more diverse socio-political constituency? Or do the terms "gay" and "queer" evoke maleness by default, thus necessitating the distinctly female term "lesbian"? Should we consider the term "lesbian" to signify a contradictory, potentially transgressive space in phallocentric symbolic regimes? Or is the postmodern move to destabilize the category of "lesbian" politically dangerous, since it threatens lesbian integrity and political viability at a time when we are still fighting for our basic human rights?[2]

Part of the reason for such passionate discussion among lesbians about definitional boundaries is that "lesbian" is such an inherently unstable category. If one false move (one "wrong" sexual partner) can define you out of existence, if the wolf is constantly howling at the door trying to deny your rights, safety, and family, if people are always asking which one of you is the man and which one is the woman, if that bungee cord in the closet keeps pulling you back in despite your best efforts to be out, and even other lesbians try to convince you that you do not exist, you can see where you might get a little twitchy about who you are.

Given all these unanswered and (for me) unanswerable questions, I propose the following as a working definition of lesbian: A lesbian is 1) a woman whose primary emotional, spiritual, and erotic connections (desires and/or activities) are with other women; and/or 2) any woman who identifies herself as a lesbian. This definition will not satisfy everyone, but it seems sufficiently inclusive that those who want to will probably be able to find themselves in it, without being so sweeping that the term loses all meaning.

Alternative Insemination

What to call insemination practices is still undecided. "Artificial insemination" (also abbreviated as "AI") is the current standard name for the procedure and enjoys wide use in medicine, law, the media, and popular conversation. "Artificial insemination by donor" (AID) is a variation introduced into the lexicon of infertility medicine in the 1950s to differentiate semen purchased from a stranger from that of the woman's husband (AIH) or male partner.[3]

Lesbians have rejected these descriptors for a variety of reasons. Many do not like the implication that "artificial" insemination is second-best to the "natural" way. Others feel the term has a technological ring that suggests human engineering. Still others object that the term disguises the natural process of conception, pregnancy, and birth once the sperm are present.[4] Women looking for less offensive language have coined such terms as "donor insemination,"[5] "alternative insemination,"[6] "alternative fertilization,"[7] and "self-insemination,"[8] in an effort to destigmatize their children's origins, and help discursively—and thereby culturally—to level the normative method of impregnation with their own. "Self-insemination," or "SI," captures more closely the procreative (and thus to some degree political) autonomy of many inseminating lesbians, but so many lesbians are involved with the infertility industry that the term does not apply to all lesbian AI. "Donor insemination" or "DI" now appears in some mainstream medical publications, suggesting that at least some acceptance of the criticisms of "artificial insemination" has spread beyond lesbian and feminist literature.[9]

While no term is perfect, I prefer "alternative insemination," or "AI," for a number of reasons. I also find the term "artificial," when attached to insemination, to be pejorative. It seems unduly naturalizing and valorizing of (hetero)sexual conception.

The term "alternative" comes from the roots "alter" and "native," which literally mean "different birth." Since lesbian AI helps to birth not only babies, but also different kinds of families, this language is apt. Further, as lesbian insemination itself is diverse, the term "alternative" points to the plurality of practices and meanings signified by AI.

Using the initials "AI" allows more flexibility for people to invent their own meanings while still using a common signifier. The "A" in "AI" could refer not only to "artificial" or "alternative" but also to "assisted" or even "artful." The "I" could mean things other than "insemination" (e.g., "impregnation").

Sperm Donor

The word "donation" has a nice ring. It implies generosity, largesse. A sperm donor, by extension, is a benevolent man, like an organ donor or a philanthropist, who bestows a gift of sperm on a hapless infertile couple. Yet in most instances "sperm donors" do not "donate" anything. "Sperm donation" is a commercial transaction in which a man sells his semen in exchange for both cash and legal immunity from parental obligations.

For these reasons, some have suggested that "sperm vendor" is a more accurate term.[10] (Other terms to describe men who provide sperm, such as "biological father," "genitor," and "ejaculatory father," are equally loaded with values and implications.) That not all sperm donors do so out of altruism does not mean sperm selling is bad, or that sperm donors are anything less than decent human beings, or that the sale of semen should be condemned. It simply means that "donor" and "donation" are misnomers. The term "sperm bank" is also a euphemism, as "sperm banks" are much more akin to retail stores than to financial institutions. "Sperm provider" (or "semen provider") has been suggested as a term that leaves open the question of motivation. A sperm provider may be a donor who gives altruistically, or a vendor who sells his sperm. Or he may have other motivations (such as wanting to test his fertility, or wanting to procreate).[11] However, "provider" has more paternal undertones than are accurate for many donors (as in "a good provider"). Further, the term "provider" typically refers to medical caregivers (as in "primary health care provider").

Perhaps part of the problem is that we need a number of new terms. Jenifer Firestone, director of Alternative Family Matters, believes that we need new language to describe the new realities of lesbian motherhood and sperm donor fatherhood, particularly for known donors (many of whom are gay men).

> [M]en who donate sperm [to lesbians] have done so in the context of various levels of involvement with their child(ren). Yet we still have only two words, *donor* and *dad,* and they do not reflect the actual relationship between the child and the man. Nor do they describe the relationship between the man and the women who used his sperm. . . . If he is not a custodial dad but is more than a known donor with no ongoing involvement, doesn't he deserve a noun of his own?[12]

I join Firestone in calling on the linguists and other creative folks among us to "have a field day" and invent new words to describe and honor these relationships. Until that happens, however, I am resigned to use "sperm donor," the most inclusive term we have. I want to emphasize, however, that donor roles—from an anonymous sperm vendor to an involved co-parent—are very diverse, and generally negotiated with great care before the AI is undertaken.

Contractual and Technological Procreation

I sometimes use this term to refer to what is otherwise known as "assisted reproductive technology" or ART, because I am concerned about the connotations of the usual terms. The phrase "reproductive technology" is suffused with industrial and patriarchal values. It implies that someone is being "reproduced," that is, replicated, perhaps on an assembly line, a la *Brave New World,* or by way of computer chip.[13] Sociologist Barbara Katz Rothman favors the term "procreative technology" because "procreation" is part of a non-commodified discourse about pregnancy, mothers, and babies.[14] I agree, yet also want to emphasize that *commercialization* of procreation is just as central to the proliferation of these practices as whatever medical technologies are used.

My solution is to use the accurate but inelegant term *contractual and technological procreation* when it does not seem too obtrusive, but to fall back on *reproductive technology* or even *ART* when it seems necessary. The actual forms of contractual and technological procreation can be broken down into three categories.[15] First we have *Contraceptive Technologies,* such as:

Birth control pills
Intrauterine devices
Norplant
Barrier methods of contraception (e.g., diaphragms)
Various methods of abortion
The "morning-after" pill

We also have *Gestational and Birth Technologies,* including:

Fetal monitoring during birth
Amniocentesis
Gestational ultrasonography
Anesthesia for labor
Vacuum birth technology
Labor-inducing and labor-slowing medicines
Cesarean sections
Surrogate motherhood

Finally we come to *Conceptive Technologies.* These are what we usually think of as reproductive technologies. Conceptive technologies include:

Alternative insemination (sperm is introduced non-coitally into a woman's
    vagina for the purpose of impregnation)
Biochemical-assisted hatching (assisted hatching, the thinning or dissection of a
    small area of the outer covering of the human egg; usually used in older
    women undergoing infertility treatment)
Blastocyst culture of embryos (embryos are cultured to the eight-cell stage or
    greater and transferred on day five of development)
Construction of artificial gametes (reprogramming somatic cells to produce arti-
    ficial gametes; this is popularly known as cloning)
Cryopreservation techniques (sperm and embryos stored at below-freezing tem-
    peratures. These techniques are used primarily on sperm. They have been
    used to freeze mouse eggs, but have not yet been successful with human eggs)
Cytoplasmic transfer (normal cytoplasm—portion of the egg surrounding the
    nucleus that is responsible for energizing the egg—from a donor egg is in-
    jected into a deficient egg)
Embryonic stem cells (human embryos and fetal stem cells developed in the lab-
    oratory may have the potential to be reprogrammed and to regenerate all tis-

sues in the body, which would have profound ramifications for gene therapy and organ transplantation)

In vitro fertilization (IVF) (embryos are typically transferred to the uterus two to three days after development in the laboratory or at the two- to eight-cell stage)

In vitro maturation of human eggs (rather than stimulate women with ovulation-inducing drugs, immature egg follicles are obtained and matured in the laboratory)

Intracytoplasmic sperm injection (ICSI) (a single sperm is injected into a harvested egg, which is then implanted into the donor's—or another woman's—uterus)

Oocyte nuclear transfer (the nucleus of the egg from the woman in treatment is removed and transplanted into an enucleated donor egg; however, reconstructed human eggs have not been successfully fertilized nor implanted into a human)

Feminism

I am a feminist and this is a feminist work. Since feminism means so many different things to different people, feminist and anti-feminist, I want to try to define "the collection of differences that can be found under the sign of feminism."[16] As a teacher of Women's Studies, I often start a new class with a discussion of feminism. I try to involve the students in defining it for themselves, to engage them with the complex politics of the term.

I have three favorite quotations that encapsulate my view of feminism. The first comes from the first Women's Studies course I ever took, as an undergraduate at the University of California at Santa Cruz in 1982. Our professor, Bettina Aptheker, told us that:

> Feminism is the collective empowerment of women as autonomous, independent [and interdependent] human beings, who shall have at *least* as much to say as men about *everything* in the arrangement of human affairs. [Emphasis is Aptheker's.][17]

This definition is sweeping yet succinct, and it includes an understanding of feminism as both empowerment and activism. I have added *interdependence* to Aptheker's independence and autonomy, to emphasize feminism's recognition of the human/natural life cycle as well as the importance of care and care giving.

The second quotation is from a speech made by suffragist Anna Julia Cooper in 1892:

> Let woman's claim be as broad in the concrete as in the abstract. We take our stand on the solidarity of humanity, the oneness of life, and the unnaturalness and injustice of all special favoritism, whether of sex, race, country or condition. We want . . . to go . . . demanding an entrance not through a gateway for our-

selves, our race, our sex or our sect, but a grand highway for humanity . . . Not until then is woman's cause won![18]

This quotation expresses the intersectionality and the utopianism of feminism, despite its complex and far from perfectly realized history, which was already well known at the time of Cooper's speech.

Finally, it is hard to resist the enduring appeal of Rebecca West's definition:

> I myself have never been able to find out precisely what feminism is; I only know that people call me a feminist whenever I express sentiments that differentiate me from a doormat.[19]

I use the term *feminism* instead of the more trendy *feminisms,* because I believe that feminism is already plural: multidimensional, transnational, and radically diverse. Feminism works toward women's equality with men and with each other, as well as celebrating and promoting women's uniqueness from men and from each other. It can stand on its own, without needing to be pluralized with an "s."

It is important to note that while significant overlaps exist between lesbianism and feminism, particularly when theorizing lesbian AI, the two categories remain analytically distinct. Lesbian choices are not necessarily feminist choices, and feminist politics do not always support the needs of lesbians.[20] Still, as the body of works to be found under the sign of "lesbian-feminism" shows, the fertile overlappings are far from incidental. Specifically lesbian feminism has been crucial to the development and gains of many branches of feminism globally. Therefore, I attempt to maintain the distinction between feminism, an ideology and politics based on valuing women, and lesbian existence, which is defined by the primacy of erotic and affective ties among women for other women.

Notes

Preface

1. By "medical establishment" I mean both mainstream and alternative medical and health systems. In the mainstream medical establishment, I include:

Personnel (doctors, nurses, physician's assistants, physical therapists, occupational therapists, and other allied health care providers)
Architecture (hospital buildings, clinics, and private physicians' offices)
Education (medical and nursing schools, schools of psychology)
Bureaucracy (HMOs and governmental regulatory agencies)
Pharmacology (pharmaceutical companies, pharmaceutical marketers, pharmacies, pharmacists)
Technology (producers of machinery and diagnostic technology such as X-rays, CAT scans, mammograms, speculums, centrifuges, chemicals, syringes, autoclaves, ovulation-predictor kits)
Mental health (psychologists, psychiatrists, marriage, family, and child counselors, social workers, art therapists)
Expertise (health educators, health policy makers, medical anthropologists and sociologists)
Legality (health lawyers and policy makers)

The holistic health/medical establishment exists parallel to the mainstream one. It includes:

What was previously known as "alternative therapy" (chiropractic, acupuncture, massage therapy, energy and spiritual healing)
Nutrition (vitamins, herbal pills, tinctures and teas, homeopathic remedies)

Fitness (home exercise equipment, gym memberships, yoga studios, exercise clothing)

In some ways, the boundaries between the mainstream medical establishment and the holistic health/medical establishment have blurred in recent years.

2. Heterosexism is the "system of advantages bestowed upon heterosexuals (especially males) that denies, denigrates, and stigmatizes any non-heterosexual form of behavior, identity, relationship, or culture. . . . [It includes the] assumption that all persons are, or should be, heterosexual and therefore excludes the needs, concerns and life experiences of persons who are gay. . . . [The use of this] term highlights parallels between antigay sentiment and other forms of prejudice, such as racism, anti-Semitism, and sexism" (Woolf 2002). The use of the terms "heterosexism" and "heterosexist" should not be construed to mean that heterosexuals are sexist people, or that sexism is somehow inherent in heterosexuality.

3. The Sperm Bank of California (TSBC), established in 1982, was the first sperm bank in the world to openly serve lesbians and single women. Of course, private physicians could order sperm from other banks at their discretion.

4. McKinlay and Arches 1985; McKinlay and Stoeckle 2001 [1988].

5. The quarantine process necessitates that the donor take an HIV test at the time he makes his sperm donation. The sperm is then frozen for six months, at which time the donor is re-tested for HIV. If his results remain negative, the sperm is released for insemination. This quarantine protects against cases where the donor has been exposed to HIV but has not had it in his system long enough to be detected on the HIV test. If the sperm were not stored until the second test, the sperm of a newly infected donor could transmit HIV to the recipient (and possibly her baby).

6. Feminists have debated the history, impact, definitions, and scope of patriarchy since the 1970s. Patriarchy was a central concept in radical, second-wave feminism of North America, Europe, and Australia, and has been developed by women beyond these regions as well. The term fell out of favor in the 1980s as analyses focused on "gender" became ascendant in feminist theory. By using the term "patriarchy," I do not mean to suggest that there is a single, global and ahistorical system under which all men oppress all women for all time and in all places. Nor do I mean that the oppression of women is the primary form of domination. Rather, I use "patriarchy" to refer to those ways in which fathers and fatherhood are valorized and empowered relative to mothers and motherhood. I use the term "patriarchal" to refer to systems in which men have legal power over mothers and children, where descent and naming are figured through the male line, and where men hold disproportionate power over women and children of their particular culture, class, religion, or other social group.

7. E.g., Bruhl 2000/2001.

8. Lasker 1998: 18, 27.

9. Ibid.: 7.

10. I use the term "ultramodern" in addition to the more popular "postmodern" because I have yet to be persuaded that we are past modernity and modernism. Rather, it seems to me that we find ourselves in an intensified modernity. Sociologist Stephen Pfohl attempts to define ultramodernity in a rhetoric that is itself ultramodern:

> The term ultramodernity connotes the omnipresence of technologically mediated rituals whereby inFORMational forms of power operate as telecommunicative substitutes for a more vulnerable ceremonial organization of bodily perception and economic moral demands. [1992: 16; capitalization is Pfohl's.]

My thinking about ultramodernity is indebted to scholars such as Zillah Eisenstein (1998), Jean Baudrillard (1988), and especially Stephen Pfohl (1992).

11. The rise of digital-based technologies also entails the globalization of markets, the flow of legal and illegal commodities: immigrant, refugee, and trafficked people, viruses, weaponry, ideas, scientific enterprise, "white noise," music, television, videos, pornography, "ethnic" food, political movements and conspiracies. In short, all kinds of good and bad things, but speeded up, turned into information, disseminated, and made profitable at unfathomably fast speeds.

12. For example, as I write this (June 2003), an appeals court in Ontario, Canada, has just mandated the legalization of marriage for same-sex couples in that province, and the city of Toronto has issued the first marriage license to a same-sex couple in North America. In Durban, South Africa, it seems likely that two lesbians—one of whom contributed eggs, the other of whom gestated and gave birth—will be deemed the legal, *and biological,* parents of their twin girls. And in Massachusetts, we await the ruling of the state's high court on legalizing marriage for same-sex couples. Unfortunately, apart from this brief mention, I am unable to incorporate these or any subsequent developments into this work.

13. E.g., Patterson 1992.

14. Chambers 1996.

15. For an interesting sociological overview of the research on lesbian and gay parents, see Stacey and Biblarz (2001).

16. I do not mean this to be disrespectful in any way toward my colleagues who do ethnographic or other empirical research on these, or related, issues. Good ethnographic research contributes to the struggle for human (e.g., legal, medical, housing, custody) rights for lesbian and gay families and family members of all stripes. Antihomophobic scholarly work across the disciplines has a cumulative impact on the lives of lesbian family members.

17. See also MacKinnon 1996.

18. Robson 1998: 19.

19. Vizenor 1990.

Chapter 1: Introduction

1. The root of the word "radical" is the same as the word "root" (and "radish"). "Radical" refers to making changes that go to the root of the problem. In activism, it means causing upheaval to the entire system and social structure. In ideas, it means challenging the root structures of the ideas.

2. Sexism is a system of power in which people who are categorized as male receive certain rights and privileges (including the right to a woman) while people who are categorized as female are restricted. Sexism includes prejudice and discrimination based on sex, as well as behavior, conditions, and attitudes that foster stereotypes or social roles based on sex (Woolf 2002). An act, or a person, is sexist if it stems from or enforces sexism.

3. I use the term "heteropatriarchy" frequently in this book because it is a heavy lifter. It points to the symbiosis between patriarchy and heterosexuality, in which both are made to seem like the "natural" order. It suggests the conjunction among heterosexuality, maleness, masculinity, and power. And it "draws attention to areas where these currently oppressive forces intersect one another, reinforce each other, and function together" (Woolf 2002). Use of the terms "heteropatriarchy" and "heteropatriarchal" should not be construed to mean that heterosexuality is patriarchal by definition, or that there is something inherently patriarchal about heterosexual relationships or sexuality.

4. "Heteronormativity denotes the equation of humanity with heterosexuality and describes the formal and informal social organization of sexuality in Western societies" (Mamo 2002: 5, cf. 3). Heteronormativity involves rigid mandates regarding marriage and reproduction and the stigmatization of non-heterosexuals. For more on heteronormativity, please see Warner (1993) and Seidman (1997).

5. I use the term "intentional lesbian families" to describe families in which a lesbian, or a lesbian couple, bear or adopt children, generally with the use of AI. This differentiates them from lesbians who have children from former heterosexual unions. It is a nicer term than "lesbian AI families," which puts too much emphasis on the process of insemination relative to everything else about the family.

6. The rights of families and the rights of family members are usually presumed to be the same, when actually they are often different and come into conflict. As I discuss later, "family rights" is often code for fathers' rights.

7. See <http://www.spermbankdirectory.com>, accessed 4 June 2003.

8. U.S. Congress 1988: 15. It appears that 1987 was the last year that any federal agency attempted to track the practice of AI, whether through counting (newborn) heads or recording the profits of the semen-banking industry.

9. Daniels and Haimes 1998: 2.

10. U.S. Congress, 1988: 10.

11. Daniels and Haimes 1998.

12. A conservative estimate of AI births is 30,000 per year in the United States alone.

Thirty thousand times fifteen years equals 450,000 births. If we estimate liberally (e.g., 65,000 per year), the numbers quickly double.

13. Barlet and Penney 1994. Sperm that has been frozen, however, whether for commercial purposes or in a quarantine process after which the donor is re-tested for HIV, is much more easily sold than fresh sperm. It can be labeled, banked, transported, and used with relative convenience. Fresh semen, by contrast, requires the cumbersome coordination of schedules among donor, recipient, and any partners, physicians, go-betweens, or other involved parties. The donor's ejaculation must be coordinated with the recipient's fertile time, often in the early morning before both go to work. Ideally, the donor will also have refrained from ejaculation in the twenty-four-hour period preceding the donation, so that the ejaculate has the highest possible sperm count. DiMarzo et al. 1990.

14. For an exploration of the psychological effects of such secrecy and lies on the children conceived through AI, see Rowland (1985).

15. The states in which it is illegal for anyone except a physician to perform AI are Alabama, Alaska, California, Montana, Nevada, New Jersey, New Mexico, Washington, Wisconsin, and Wyoming.

16. Wikler 1991.

17. U.S. Congress 1988.

18. Syphilis, gonorrhea, CMV, and chlamydia can all be transmitted to the fetus in utero, but are all treatable with antibiotics, and could—and should—be cured before insemination. Herpes is not transmitted until birth, and there are even ways to avoid this. Through the 1980s, U.S. physicians would rather inseminate highly (and wrongly) stigmatized women with STDs than lesbians.

19. Stern et al. 2001.

20. Jacob, Klock, and Maier 1999.

21. States that mandate sealing AI records are Alabama, Arkansas, Connecticut, Idaho, Illinois, Kansas, Minnesota, Missouri, Montana, Nevada, New Jersey, New Mexico, New York, Ohio, Oregon, Washington, and Wisconsin.

22. During this period, lesbians far less frequently declared themselves "married," even when in long-term couples (Sherman 1992).

23. Obviously, lesbians who inseminate outside of the medical context do not literally "self-inseminate" since a man's sperm is necessary. In theory, human reproductive cloning could change this fact.

24. Stacey 1996: 7.

25. 478 U.S. 186 [1986].

26. Kaplan and Squier 1999.

27. Pollitt 1996.

28. Stacey and Davenport 2002: 357.

29. Stacey 1996: 45–48.

30. Stacey and Davenport 2002: 357.

31. Alexander 1991: 146.

32. Eaton 1995: 69.
33. Foucault 1990 [1976].
34. Blank 1998.
35. Rich 1979 [1977].
36. Curie-Cohen 1979.
37. Norsigian 1976.
38. Leiblum et al. 1995.
39. Of course, not all families with men in them are patriarchal.
40. Chambers 1996.
41. O'Hanlan 1995: 102.
42. U.S. Congress 1988: 23.
43. The physicians in the OTA study answered (as follows) the question "What proportion of the patients who have requested artificial insemination in the past year were":

> Married couples: 92.2%
> Women without a partner: 2.9%
> Unmarried couples (heterosexual): 2.2%
> Unmarried couples (lesbian): 0.7%
> Do not know marital status: 0.7% (U.S. Congress 1988: 23).

44. It would require a different kind of research to try to identify this population, research that seems unlikely to find funding in the current political climate.
45. E.g., Benkoff 1994; Martin 1993.
46. E.g., Harvard Law School 1990; Rosenbloom 1996. Differences with bisexual and transgender people are de-emphasized as well.
47. E.g., Lewin 1993; Pepper 1999.
48. E.g., Corea 1985; Farquhar 1996; Robertson 1994; Stanworth 1987.
49. E.g., Mattes 1994; Noble 1987.
50. Daniels and Haimes 1998.
51. Franklin 1992: 128.

Chapter 2: Setting the Historical Stage

1. Latour 1993.
2. It is beyond the scope of this book to engage in major debates over periodization. It does bear mentioning, however, that the terms "ultramodern" (Pfohl 1992) and "modernist" (Lash 1990) are strong contenders to replace the term "postmodern."
3. Rothman 1989.
4. It seems that the symbolism of the fetus as the seed of the man growing in the woman's body still has a great deal of power, as is evidenced by the discourse and political power of the anti-abortion movement.
5. O'Brien 1981: 48.

6. Juliet Flower MacCannell (1991) argues that rather than revering and obeying old men, modern males gain power through "old boy" networks, fraternal societies, and other (hierarchical) bonds with male peers and buddies.
7. Stacey 1996: 7.
8. Ibid.: 7–8.
9. Kahn 2000: 163; cf. Strathern 1992; Franklin 1992.
10. Kahn 2000: 163–64; Franklin 1995.
11. Foucault 1990 [1975]: 144.
12. O'Brien 1981.
13. This is, of course, a reference to the important socialist-feminist essay "The Un-happy Marriage of Marxism and Feminism: Towards a More Progressive Union" (Bridges and Hartmann 1981).
14. See Hansen and Philipson (1990) for a comprehensive investigation of socialist-feminism.
15. E.g., Gilman 1966 [1898]; Holmstrom 2002.
16. For more on the relationship of capitalism and patriarchy, the anthology *Women, Class, and the Feminist Imagination* (Hansen and Philipson 1990) is an excellent place to start.
17. Sperm-as-sacred-seed-of-life is sometimes known as "Spermocracy."
18. Schmidt and Moore 1998: 18–19.
19. For Max Weber, one of the fathers of sociology, disenchantment was a core characteristic of modernity.
20. In Pfeffer 1987: 94.
21. This was before the emergence of lesbian AI. Pfeffer 1987: 94.
22. Harlow 1996: 184.
23. Blankenhorn 1995: 184.
24. See Ibid.: chapter 9, "The Sperm Father."
25. Ibid.: 184.
26. Ibid.: 182.
27. Radin 1996.
28. Farquhar 1996: 3. Animal husbandry is the primary site of AI in the United States. Factory farming industries are dependent on AI and other forms of procreative technology such as "egg flushing." Procreative technologies are often used on non-human animals before they are approved for human use. For truly troubling descriptions of the standard abuses of captive "farm" animals via procreative technologies see Corea (1985).
29. For more feminist analyses of technoscience, please see Haraway (1997) and Clarke and Olesen (1999).
30. I put "civilized" in quotes since non-human animals tend to possess more of the virtues of civilization than humans do.
31. The Catholic Church has condemned AI using non-husband semen because it involves at least two sins: masturbation on the part of the donor and adultery on the

part of the woman. However, with the use of a special semen collection device (SCD) used during "normal intercourse," a husband's semen may be used for AI. Not surprisingly, numerous fertility clinics offer said devices and instructions as to their use.

32. Englert 1994.
33. O'Brien 1981: 48.
34. See Theweleit, 1987 [1977].
35. Watney 1990.
36. For example, in 1997, conservative Christian leader Jerry Falwell publicly referred to lesbian comedian Ellen Degeneres as "Ellen Degenerate."
37. Gibson 1997: 125.
38. "Homophobia" is a problematic term. Literally, it refers to an irrational fear or hatred of homosexuals and homosexuality, as well as any actions based on that fear or hatred (e.g., lesbian bashing). One reason to avoid the term "homophobia" is that it tends to imply that the oppression of LGBT people is individual and psychopathological, rather than normative and systematic. For more on "homophobia," see Teish 1985.
39. Theweleit 1987; Theweleit 1989.
40. For example, see the Donor Catalogues from California Cryobank (2003b), Fairfax Cryobank (2002), or the Sperm Bank of California (2003).
41. Leiblum et al. 1995.
42. See California Cryobank (2003c) for example.
43. American Society for Reproductive Medicine 2001a.
44. Genetics and IVF Institute 2002.
45. California Cryobank, Inc. 2002.
46. California Cryobank, Inc. 1991.
47. Schmidt and Moore 1998.
48. E.g., Paul 1995.
49. California Cryobank, Inc. 2003.
50. Scandinavian Cryobank 2003.
51. Williams 1991: 226.
52. In a matriarchal society, at least in theory, one would not need to be so concerned with the physical appearance of children, because everybody would know who the child's mother is, and hence to which kinship group it belonged at birth.
53. Tsing 1990.
54. Ibid.: 296. Hence Carby's (1987) contention that oppressive stereotypes of black women were inseparable from the social control of white women.
55. Solinger 1998: 382.
56. Ibid.: 382–83.
57. Ladd-Taylor and Umansky 1998. Such norms change over time and by cultural location. White U.S. women who forswore marriage in the generations between

1780 and 1840 were valorized as "Blessedly Single, and Singly Blessed" (Chambers-Schiller 1984).

58. Haraway 1997: 30.

59. Gibson 1997: 116. Please see the discussion of degeneracy earlier in this chapter.

60. She may also fall under any of these categories depending on her biography and demographics, and on who is doing the categorizing. My point is that her situation is not easily and automatically reducible to these predominant tropes.

61. Lewin (1993: 8) attributes this observation to the ever-insightful Rayna Rapp.

62. Anzaldùa, 1990b.

Chapter 3: Disfertile Discourses

1. Mamo 2002.

2. Ibid.: 114.

3. Ehrenreich and English 1973.

4. States in which it is illegal for anyone except a licensed physician to perform AI are Alabama, Alaska, California, Colorado, Connecticut, Georgia, Idaho, Illinois, Minnesota, Montana, New Jersey, New Mexico, New York, North Carolina, Ohio, Oklahoma, Oregon, Tennessee, Texas, Virginia, Washington, Wisconsin, Wyoming (Lesbian Moms' Organization 1995).

5. E.g., Todd 1989; Saxton and Howe 1987; Conrad and Kern 1990; White 1990.

6. Zola 1990: 209.

7. Arms 1975; Wertz and Wertz 1989.

8. Foucault 1990 [1976]; Terry and Urla 1995.

9. E.g., Ehrenreich and English 1973; Hubbard 1990.

10. Zola 1990: 104.

11. Schmidt and Moore 1998.

12. Boston Women's Health Book Collective 1992: 387.

13. Santa Cruz Women's Health Collective 1979: 49.

14. Ibid.

15. Wikler 1991.

16. Jacob et al. 1999.

17. E.g., Benkov 1994; Hanscombe and Forster 1982; Pollack and Vaughn 1987; Wakeling and Bradstock 1995.

18. Numbers on self-insemination are not collected, but the lesbian grapevine indicates that self-insemination is still alive and well, although not as commonly practiced due to (realistic) fears about HIV transmission from gay male sperm donors, who were previously the first choice of many inseminating lesbians (Weston 1991).

19. Medicalized and demedicalized approaches to AI might be compared on many bases, not all of which make the medicalized practice look bad. A doctor's ability to procure fresh, anonymous sperm is sometimes superior to that of a self-inseminator

who has only her own extended social network to draw on. Frozen sperm is also more convenient, and much safer. Particularly with the risk of HIV, which has a relatively long incubation period, one can freeze a man's sperm, test him for HIV, wait six months if he is negative, test him again, and if he is still negative release the sperm. This gives the provider a chance to screen out those sperm donors who are newly infected, among which it may be too early for the HIV test to detect signs of infection. Cryotechnology also gives the provider an opportunity to build up a sperm collection, or to buy from a sperm bank, and thus to provide a greater choice of sperm donors for her clients.

20. In fact, Mamo (2002) argues that lesbian insemination today (at least in the San Francisco Bay Area) is neither low-tech nor high-tech, but something that she calls "hybrid/meso tech."
21. Mohler and Frazer 2002.
22. Ibid.: 32–33.
23. E.g., Greil 1990.
24. Whether infertility qua infertility is necessarily a medical condition, or ought to be so considered, is also debatable.
25. American Society for Reproductive Medicine. 1996–1997.
26. Boston Women's Health Book Collective 1992: 500.
27. Doyal 1995.
28. In sperm-washing, a semen sample is centrifuged (spun) to isolate the sperm, then chemically treated to enhance its likelihood of causing a pregnancy. At that point it may be frozen or inseminated directly into a woman's uterus.
29. ICSI is a form of IVF that involves hyperovulating and surgically extracting eggs from the woman's body, injecting them with a single sperm cell in a petri dish, and then, with the administration of additional hormones, inserting the fertilized egg back into the woman's body.
30. American Society for Reproductive Medicine 1996b.
31. E.g., Prager 1982.
32. Artificial insemination may be the only "treatment" in which the person treated has nothing wrong with her.
33. Daniels 1998: 177.
34. Sullivan 1997.
35. Ibid.: 84.
36. The overwhelming passage into law of the 1995 "Defense of Marriage Act" (DOMA) is but one example of the willingness of Congress to deny lesbians and gay men civil rights.
37. See discussion of the pathologization of lesbians on pages 53-54.
38. States in which health insurance providers are required to cover infertility services are Arkansas, Hawaii, Illinois, Maryland, Massachusetts, Montana, New Jersey, Ohio, Rhode Island, and West Virginia. Those in which it must be offered are California, Connecticut, and Texas.

39. Arkansas Statutes Annotated, Sections 23–85–137 and 23–86–118.
40. Conrad and Kern 1990: 227.
41. American Society for Reproductive Medicine 1996. I put quotation marks around "childbearing age" because women in this category may or may not be involved in childbearing, and need not be defined by their procreative capacities. This phrase also becomes increasingly meaningless with the progress of procreative technologies that, at least in theory, may lift the limit off of how old a woman can be and still bear a child.
42. American Society for Reproductive Medicine 1996. This is sometimes phrased inaccurately (but more impressively) as "ten million people" suffering from infertility in the United States (e.g. Hubbard 1990: 202).
43. Hubbard 1990.
44. One form of false advertising the ASRM guidelines caution against is substituting the number of fertilized eggs for the number of live births in order to inflate success rates (American Society for Reproductive Medicine 1990).
45. Ibid.
46. American Society for Reproductive Medicine 1996a. See my discussion of PIVMO (penis in vagina with male orgasm), in note 46, page 202.
47. The diagnosis "homosexuality" was removed from the DSM-III by a vote of the Board of Trustees of the American Psychiatric Association. But a variant— "ego-dystonic homosexuality"—was added in its place. See Irvine 1990: 253 and 123.
48. Duka and DeCherney 1996.
49. It bears noting that Western medicine often considers fertility (pregnancy and childbirth) to be an illness as much as infertility.
50. Duka and DeCherney 1996.
51. Resolve 2003.
52. Genesis 30:1. Quoted in Kahn 2000: 70.
53. According to the 1988 survey conducted by the Office of Technology Assessment (OTA), 52 percent of physicians who perform AI stated that they would refuse services to "unmarried" women. Fifteen percent stated that they would refuse AI services to "homosexual" women. These numbers are a bit confusing, but I take them to mean that 52 percent would refuse any unmarried women, while an additional 15 percent (or 67 percent total) would refuse insemination to lesbians (U.S. Congress 1988). See Kahn 2000: 70.
54. U.S. Congress, Office of Technology Assessment 1988. Excluding incarcerated women from such an important national survey is problematic, since institutionalized women represent a growing segment of the female citizenry, not an "exceptional" group. Incarcerated women are mothers, have families, and suffer overall from very poor health. By excluding this population from the survey, the results are skewed to present a rosier picture of U.S. women's experiences than really exists. An excellent book on women's incarceration and reproduction, in the broadest

sense of both terms, is *Policing the National Body: Race, Gender, and Criminalization* (Silliman and Bhattacharjee 2002).

55. Abma et al. 1997.
56. Ibid.
57. The medical language around AI frequently promotes lesbian invisibility (e.g. Duberman et al. 1991; Faderman 1981; Irigaray 1985b; Lorde 1984; Nestle 1987; Rich 1981). Invisibility contributes to the heterosexism endemic to patriarchal culture and political institutions. It is also part of the vicious circle of socially imposed obstacles faced by lesbians who have or want to have children.
58. Rosenbloom 1996: xiv.
59. Rosenbloom 1996.
60. Sedgwick 1990. Lesbian invisibility may be replaced by equally brutal queer hyper-visibility, but that is another question for another time.
61. Weston 1991: 5.
62. Terry 1995.
63. Katz 1995.
64. Zola 1990: 403.
65. Daly 1984: 97.
66. Ehrenreich and English 1973: 139–40.
67. Tsing 1990.
68. Sedgwick 1990.
69. Nordenberg 1997.
70. Ibid.
71. American Society for Reproductive Medicine 1997.
72. Pollock 1998.
73. Ibid.
74. Academic superstars are the exception to this rule.
75. See Foucault (1990 [1976]) for a philosophical and historical exploration of the discursive, penal, and medical "treatment" of homosexuals in the West.
76. Ibid.; Irvine 1990; e.g., Harvard Law School 1990: 139.
77. Strong and Schinfeld 1984.
78. At the time that the Strong and Schinfeld article was published (1984), and all the more so today, the "available" social science data could more accurately be characterized as strongly refuting the suggestion that lesbian parents are inferior, on any measure, to their heterosexual counterparts.
79. Ibid.
80. Mattes 1994.
81. Blank 1998.
82. This understanding is indebted to Sofia Gruskin at Harvard University School of Public Health.
83. E.g., Perkoff 1985; *Korn v. Potter.* See my discussion of the latter case later in this chapter.

84. IFFS 1995.

85. Ibid.

86. Ibid.

87. See my discussion of the "infertile couple" in chapter 3 (Disfertile Discourses).

88. Harlow 1996.

89. Jacob et al. 1999.

90. Englert 1994.

91. Jacob et al. 1999: 211.

92. While it may seem at first glance that the illegal status of lesbianism itself might be the bigger impediment to lesbian AI, such laws are rarely enforced, and are most often used to support other oppressive policies that limit the rights and freedoms of lesbians. For instance, in the United States, one does not read of lesbians being thrown in jail for being lesbians, but one does read about lesbians being denied jobs, housing, and parental rights for being lesbians.

93. U.S. Congress 1988.

94. *Korn v. Potter* (1996–04–02), British Columbia Supreme Court, A953370, available from the Canadian Legal Information Institute, <http://www.canlii.org/bc/cas/bcsc/1996bcsc10460.html>, accessed 18 July 2002.

95. Harlow 1996.

96. Ibid.: note 90.

97. Harlow 1996: note 219.

98. Some legal scholars are optimistic, however, that if statutes such as those proposed in these three states were to pass, they could be successfully challenged as unconstitutional (Harlow 1996: note 42).

99. The category "infertile couple" was constructed to help U.S. wives of Vietnam veterans have access to AI when their husbands were sterile due to combat injuries. It was a progressive move at the time, which I certainly would not want to reverse without putting something better in its place.

Chapter 4: Legal Legitimacy and the Lesbian AI "Bastard"

1. Minter 1996.

2. The church and medicine use the law to strengthen and enforce their rules. The AMA lobbied to outlaw home births, and organized religious lobbies influence local and national politics. Still, only the law can send a person to jail.

3. E.g., Arnup and Boyd 1995; Fineman 1995; Polikoff 1990.

4. E.g., Harvard Law School 1990; Minter 1996; Rich 1976.

5. For an intelligent and chilling discussion of these issues see Andrews (1999).

6. Harvard Law School 1990.

7. Marquis 2000.

8. States without any laws regulating AI are Pennsylvania, South Dakota, and Vermont. Puerto Rico and the U.S. Virgin Islands also lack AI-related statutes.

9. States with anti-discrimination statutes are California, Connecticut, Hawaii, Massachusetts, Minnesota, New Hampshire, New Jersey, Rhode Island, Vermont, and Wisconsin.

10. The states explicitly banning same-sex marriage are Alaska, Alabama, Arkansas, Arizona, California, Colorado, Florida, Georgia, Hawaii, Iowa, Idaho, Illinois, Indiana, Kansas, Kentucky, Louisiana, Maine, Michigan, Minnesota, Mississippi, Montana, North Carolina, North Dakota, Nebraska, Oklahoma, Pennsylvania, South Carolina, South Dakota, Tennessee, Texas, Utah, Virginia, Washington, and West Virginia.

11. National Gay and Lesbian Task Force n.d.

12. 18 V.S.A. § 1204 (Vermont's Civil Union Law). The full text of the law is at "Vermont Secretary of State—Civil Unions Law," <http://www.sec.state.vt.us/otherprg/civilunions/civilunionlaw.html>, accessed 5 June 2002.

13. Markowitz n.d.

14. National Gay and Lesbian Task Force n.d.

15. Baldauf 1997.

16. National Center for Lesbian Rights 2001.

17. As of August 2003, second-parent adoptions have been granted by trial court judges in: Alabama (selected counties), Alaska (Juneau), Delaware (selected counties), Hawaii (selected counties), Indiana (White County), Iowa (selected counties), Louisiana (Orleans Parish), Maryland (selected counties), Minnesota (selected counties), Nevada (selected counties), New Mexico (selected counties), Oregon (Multnomah County), Rhode Island (selected counties), Texas (selected counties), and Washington (selected counties).

Second-parent adoptions have been approved by appellate courts in California, Illinois, Indiana, Massachusetts, Pennsylvania, New York, New Jersey, Vermont, and the District of Columbia.

In 2002, the Nebraska Court of Appeals held that Nebraska must recognize a second-parent adoption granted in Pennsylvania, even though the adoption would not have been permitted in Nebraska. This is the first and thus far the only appellate decision addressing inter-state recognition of second-parent adoptions. In addition, there are statutes expressly permitting second-parent adoptions in California, Connecticut, and Vermont.

On the other hand, appellate courts in four states—Colorado, Nebraska, Ohio, and Wisconsin—have held that second-parent adoptions are not permissible under their respective adoption statutes (NCLR 2003).

18. States in which the court has ruled that state law permits second-parent adoption by same-sex couples are Alabama, Alaska, Hawaii, Indiana, Iowa, Louisiana, Maryland, Michigan, Minnesota, Nevada, New Mexico, Oregon, Rhode Island, Texas, and Washington.

19. Minter 1996: 219.

20. States in which an appellate court has ruled that state adoption law permits second-

parent adoption by same-sex couples are Illinois, Massachusetts, New York, and New Jersey.

21. States in which the adoption law explicity permits second-parent adoption by same-sex couples are California, Connecticut, and Vermont.

22. In Colorado, Nebraska, Ohio, and Wisconsin, an appellate court has ruled that state adoption law does not allow second-parent adoption by same-sex couples.

23. Sullivan 1992.

24. Gartrell et al. 2000: 547.

25. Williams 1991.

26. The following countries have enforceable laws against sex between consenting adults of the same sex: Afghanistan, Algeria, Angola, Bahrain, Bangladesh, Barbados, Benin, Bhutan, Botswana, Brunei, Burundi, Cameroon, Cape Verde, Cook Islands, Democratic Republic of Congo, Djibouti, Eritrea, Ethiopia, Fiji Islands, Gambia, Ghana, Grenada, Guyana, Guinea, India, Iran, Jamaica, Kenya, Kiribati, Kosovar Autonomous Republic, Kuwait, Laos, Lebanon, Liberia, Libya, Malawi, Malaysia, Maldives, Marshall Islands, Mauritania, Mauritius, Morocco, Mozambique, Myanmar (Burma), Namibia, Nauru, Nepal, Nicaragua, Nigeria, Niue, Oman, Pakistan, Papua New Guinea, Qatar, Russia: Chechnya, Saint Lucia, Saudi Arabia, Senegal, Seychelles, Sierra Leone, Singapore, Solomon Islands, Somalia, Sri Lanka, Sudan, Swaziland, Syria, Tajikistan, Tanzania, Togo, Tokelau, Tonga, Trinidad and Tobago, Tunisia, Turkmenistan, Tuvalu, Uganda, United Arab Emirates, Uzbekistan, Western Sahara, Western Samoa, Yemen, Zambia, Zimbabwe. IGLHRC 2003.

27. As of June 2003, Kansas, Missouri, Oklahoma, and Texas had laws banning only same-sex sodomy. Alabama, Florida, Idaho, Louisiana, Mississippi, North Carolina, South Carolina, Utah, Virginia, and Puerto Rico prohibited sodomy between both same-sex and different-sex partners.

28. Robson 1992.

29. States that define the consenting husband as the legal father are Alabama, Alaska, Arizona, Arkansas, California, Colorado, Connecticut, Georgia, Idaho, Illinois, Indiana, Kansas, Louisiana, Maine, Massachusetts, Minnesota, Mississippi, Missouri, Montana, Nevada, New Jersey, New Mexico, New York, North Carolina, North Dakota, Ohio, Oregon, Rhode Island, South Carolina, Tennessee, Utah, Washington, Wisconsin, and Wyoming.

30. States specifying inheritance rights for offspring conceived with AI are Arkansas, Connecticut, Georgia, Indiana, Montana, New York, and North Carolina. States that specify or reference child support obligations are Arizona, Arkansas, California, Georgia, Indiana, Kansas, Louisiana, Mississippi, Montana, Nebraska, New Mexico, North Dakota, Ohio, Rhode Island, South Carolina, Utah, Virginia, Wisconsin, and Wyoming.

31. States that assert the donor's lack of paternity are Alabama, California, Colorado, Connecticut, Idaho, Illinois, Minnesota, Missouri, Montana, Nevada, New Hamp-

shire, New Jersey, New Mexico, Ohio, Oregon, Washington, Wisconsin, and Wyoming. New Hampshire, New Jersey, New Mexico, and Washington stipulate that if the parties have an agreement that the donor has rights and responsibilities, he does.

32. States referencing HIV in their AI-related statues are California, Delaware, Florida, Idaho, Illinois, Indiana, Iowa, Kentucky, Louisiana, Michigan, New Hampshire, New Mexico, Ohio, Oregon, Virginia, and West Virginia.

33. States limiting the practice of AI to physicians and those supervised by them are Arkansas, Connecticut, Georgia, Idaho, Ohio, and Oregon. States that define AI as only that performed by a physician are Alabama, Alaska, California, Montana, Nevada, New Jersey, New Mexico, Washington, Wisconsin, and Wyoming.

34. States referencing lesbians in their AI statues are California, New Jersey, New York, Rhode Island, and Washington.

35. Kaiser 1987–1988. This lack of specificity has a positive side, since any law that differentiated between lesbians and others seeking AI would almost certainly be punitive.

36. Delaney 1991.

37. E.g., Minow 1991.

38. Chambers 1996.

39. Robson 1998: 171–95.

40. Hunter 1997 [1991]: 299.

41. E.g., Kendall and Haaland 1996.

42. How the family is defined is of course intimately related to sexism and heterosexism, as well as race and class.

43. Woodhouse 1993: 1783.

44. E.g., *Bennett v. Jeffreys; Ronald FF v. Cindy GG*. Woodhouse (1993) analyses these cases in detail.

45. E.g., *In re Raquel Marie X*. This case is also discussed at length in Woodhouse (1993). PIVMO is an acronym for "penis in vagina with male orgasm," coined by Canadian philosopher Kathryn Pauly Morgan and is more specific, and therefore more useful, than the more common technical term "heterosexual intercourse." Morgan explains: "This [PIVMO] is a term that I coined . . . as a shorthand way of referring to the mechanics of heterophallocentrism (personal email communication, 6/02).

The term "intercourse" is at the core of phallic narratives of sexuality, where it is considered to be at the etiological and teleological end of a strictly defined, linear progression of gestures that exhaust the definition of "sex." One of the more offensive of the prior terms integral to the "intercourse" discourse is "foreplay," an umbrella term that is meant to "include" (and thus devalue) every sexual activity other than penile-vaginal intercourse. In addition to being irredeemably heterosexist, this discourse is part of a Freudian-derived social control system that pressures women (and men) to engage in penile-vaginal intercourse as a precondition to the achievement of sexual adulthood. That the word "sex" is used interchangeably with "intercourse," and that "intercourse" is widely assumed to mean penile-vaginal intercourse, is a reflection of the insidious (in this case discursive) heterosexism in our lives.

This phallocentric discourse of sexuality is written into law. Ruthann Robson elaborates, "There is a violence in the legal text of our sexuality [statutes criminalizing lesbian sexual expression] that would describe any activities within our lovemaking as "deviate," as "perverted," as "unnatural," or even with reference to words like intercourse or copulation (1992: 47)." Since it presumably does not involve PIVMO, the male authors of such legal texts find lesbian sexuality either invisible or appalling. (It is interesting to note that rape within marriage was not defined as problematic at all).

Morgan developed the concept of PIVMO in relation to Karen Rotkin's article, "The Phallacy of our Sexual Norm" (1976 [1972]). She also discusses it in "The Moral Politics of Sex Education" (Morgan 1996).

46. Rosenbloom 1996.
47. National Center for Lesbian Rights 2003.
48. Ibid.
49. International Gay and Lesbian Task Force 1998.
50. Quebec 2002: 538.1.
51. Quebec 2002: 538.3.
52. Quebec 2002: 538.2.
53. Quebec 2002: 539.
54. Quebec 2002: 521.18.
55. Lieden University Law professor Kees Waaldijk has helpfully provided both his translation of the "Dutch Law on the opening up of marriage for same-sex partners (plus explanatory memorandum)" (<http://ruljis.liedenuniv.nl./user/cwaaldi/www/NHR/transl-marr.html>) and the "Dutch law on the opening up of adoption for same-sex partners (plus explanatory memorandum)" (<http://ruljis.liedenuniv.nl./user/cwaaldi/www/NHR/transl-adop.html>). He also has an English-language page of updates on same-sex marriage in the Netherlands, which includes statistics on how many have registered and more (<http://rulj287. leidenuniv.nl/user/cwaaldij/www/NHR/news.htm>). Sites accessed 6 July 2002. All information about the Netherlands in these paragraphs comes from these sources.
56. Fineman Thomadsen 1991: 281.
57. E.g., Mossman 1991.
58. Ross 1996.
59. Bartlett and Kennedy 1991.
60. E.g., Minow 1993.
61. Burnham 1993 [1987]; Cleaver 1997.

62. Bartlett and Kennedy 1991: 2.

63. Doane and Hodges 1987. Doane and Hodges develop the notion that nostalgic texts are those that strive to undermine feminism by reasserting the permanence of a stable referent against the heteroglossia of women's voices. Interestingly, this stable referent usually ends up being the Mother in the heteropatriarchal family, whom the nostalgic author seeks to establish as timeless and natural.

64. Stychin and Herman 1995: xi.

65. Rosenbloom 1996.

66. Twenty-eight states have AI statutes. Only seven refer to unmarried women (Harvard Law School 1990: 143).

67. Kaiser 1987–1988: 796.

68. Minow 1991: 271.

69. Harvard Law School 1990: 140.

70. Ibid.

71. Ibid.: 143. This protection from intrusion by the sperm donor for married women is of course only guaranteed in the twenty-eight states that have statutes governing AI.

72. An interesting side note is that Mary and Victoria had split up by this point, and Victoria, while denied "de facto parent" status, was granted visitation rights (Kaiser 1987–1988: 800–801). This decision of the court to grant visitation rights to Victoria in the *Jhordan C.* case, considering the fact that as non-biological mother she had no standing before the court, was idiosyncratic, to say the least.

73. Polikoff 1990. The theory of the de facto parent was first applied in 1973 in a case that, as far as we know, was unrelated to lesbians. "We use the term 'de facto parent' to refer to that person who, on a day-to-day basis, assumes the role of parent, seeking to fulfill both the child's physical needs and his [sic] psychological needs for affection and care" (Shapiro and Schultz 1985–1986: 273, citing Goldstein, Freud, and Solnit [1973]).

74. Macdonald 1992. I put "surrogate" in quotations because the "surrogate" mother *is* the mother (unless and until she relinquishes her child for adoption). "Surrogacy" is a term of art that hides that fact and can distort our understanding. The same is true of sexual "surrogates."

75. Chambers 1996.

76. The ACLU wrote this in a 1994 amicus brief in support of a lesbian family against paternity claims by their sperm donor. Quoted in Polikoff 1996: 387–88.

77. Ibid.

78. Delaney 1991: 181.

79. Reinfeld 2000.

80. Tsing 1990.

81. Williams 1995: 8–9.

82. Ibid.

83. Weston 1991: 170.

84. E.g., Ehrenreich and English 1973.
85. Sedgwick 1990: 94.
86. Many mainstream religious denominations today embrace or are tolerant of lesbian families, while others maintain their historic antagonism.
87. This sense that lesbians and gay men are "unnatural" is central to the rejection of equal rights for lesbians and gay men in the non-Western world. For a lucid exploration of the reluctance of people in various cultures to accept gay and lesbian rights, see Howard-Hassman (2001).
88. Rosenbloom 1996: xxvi.
89. Stacey 1996: 6.
90. Ernulf et al. 1989.
91. Again, families and family members are overlapping but not identical categories.

Chapter 5: The Economics of Lesbian Insemination

1. Colen (1989) first articulated the concept of stratified reproduction. She used it to describe the social forces that encourage privileged women to reproduce while punishing other groups for reproducing. Numerous authors have since developed the idea of stratified reproduction.
2. Patterson 1995.
3. Baran and Pannor 1989.
4. "The National Survey of Family Growth (NSFG), sponsored by the National Center for Health Statistics, United States Department of Health and Human Services, is a multipurpose survey based on personal interviews with a national sample of women 15–44 years of age in the civilian noninstitutionalized population of the United States. Its main function is to collect data on factors affecting pregnancy and women's health in the United States. . . . Topics covered in the series include the number of children women have had and the number they expect to have in the future, intended and unintended births, first sexual intercourse and partners, marriage, cohabitation, impaired fecundity, sterilization operations, breastfeeding, maternity leave, child care, adoption, stepchildren, foster children, health insurance coverage, family planning, and health conditions and behavior, including smoking. . . . HIV testing, pelvic inflammatory disease, and sex education" (Inter-University Consortium for Political and Social Research 2002).
5. While married childless women are ten times as likely as an unmarried childless woman to make an infertility visit, they are thirteen times as likely to receive advice, seventeen times as likely to receive tests (on the man or woman), twenty times as likely to receive ovulation drugs, twenty times as likely to receive surgery or treatment for blocked tubes, and a staggering forty-seven times as likely to receive ART (Abma et al. 1997: 65, table 55).
6. Ibid.

7. Just shy of 20 percent of women with just high school (or GED) and 19.4 percent of women with some college got "any services" as compared to 18 percent of women with a bachelor's degree or higher.

8. Ibid. The exact figures are bachelor's degree or higher: 2.2 percent; some college: 1.2 percent; high school education: 1.1 percent; no high school diploma: 0.2 percent.

9. Ibid.

10. See the discussion on quantifying lesbian AI in appendix A.

11. While AI is more expensive than PIVMO, it is inexpensive for a reproductive technology, and it is less expensive than adoption.

12. The sperm banks that are known to serve the lesbian community are the Sperm Bank of California, Pacific Reproductive Services, and Rainbow Flag Health Services. Those listed on the first page of an internet search were California Cryobank, Xytex, and the Sperm Bank of New York, in addition to some of those listed above.

13. Pepper 1999.

14. Remember, the ASRM has asserted that there is no proven way to preselect semen to influence the sex of the offspring (American Society for Reproductive Medicine 2001a).

15. Macaulay et al. 1995.

16. Nachtigall 1994.

17. Wortley et al. 1998.

18. Nachtigall 1994.

19. Carrington 1999.

20. Ibid.: 210–11.

21. Mamo 2002.

22. Carrington 1999.

23. Robson 1998: 30.

24. O'Hanlan 1995.

25. French feminist theorists of the May '68 generation articulated the meaning and function of fluids, as opposed to solids, in Western culture (e.g. Cixous 1976 [1975]; Irigaray 1985a), as have other critics and philosophers (e.g. Theweleit 1987 [1977]). All explored liquids, fluids, flux, and flow as signifying a "feminine" threat to phallic symbolic structures.

26. To reify literally means to consider an abstract concept to be real. I use it in the Marxian sense of investing something unreal with reality, solidity, and permanence, usually so it can be bought and sold.

27. American Society for Reproductive Medicine 1997.

28. Pfohl 1992.

29. Thanks to Anne Pollock for reminding me of this fact (personal communication, 13 August 2002).

30. Anne Pollock points out that this is even more true for egg donation, where consumers expect still more "value" because of their high financial investment (personal communication, 13 August 2002).

31. Hitchens 1985.
32. Legal scholar Ruth Colker (1996) makes the intriguing argument that women are not only economically poorer then men after divorce, but also reproductively "poorer." Because men's sperm is generally so abundant, she argues, they have many more opportunities to make children than do women. One of her conclusions is that women should almost always be given control of any contested frozen "embryos" at the time of divorce.
33. I use the term "liquid classes" to refer to the upper-middle class and above, who valorize being financially liquid, physically flexible, lean, psychologically resilient, and mentally agile. For more about ultramodernity's overvaluing of liquidity, see Martin (1999) and Pfohl (1992).
34. Some sperm banks now offer customers the option of storing sperm from a single donor for multiple inseminations. Some lesbians use this option to create a biogenetic tie between their children when each woman in the couple births an AI baby.
35. Engels 1963 [1884]: 38.
36. Daniels 1998.
37. O'Brien 1981: 54.
38. Ehrenreich 1983. Many feminist scholars have noted that individualism is inherently masculinist. As Sarah Franklin observes, "The very term 'individual,' meaning *one who cannot be divided,* can only mean the male, as it is precisely the process of one individual becoming two which occurs through a woman's pregnancy. Pregnancy is precisely about one body becoming two bodies, two bodies, becoming one, the exact antithesis of individuality" (Franklin 1992: 203). Valerie Hartouni also re produced this quotation in her essay "A Study in Reproductive Technologies" (1999: 264, cf. 11). This ability of women to "be divided" is a biological difference between the sexes regardless of whether a woman ever chooses to become pregnant.
39. E.g., Kovacs et al. 1983; Lui et al. 1995; Sauer et al. 1989. A thoughtful exception to this trend is Rowland (1983). For a summary and discussion of existing research, see Daniels and Haimes (1998).
40. Daniels 1998: 82.
41. Ibid.: 89.
42. Ibid.
43. Ibid.: 90.
44. Ibid.: 91.
45. This is a primary reason that the Catholic Church is against AI (except for certain highly ritualized forms of AIH), just as it is against birth control and other conceptive technologies.
46. Of course, a woman who wanted a baby could always go out and find a man to impregnate her "the old fashioned way." Yet the potential social stigmatization that might result for unmarried woman was often prohibitive.
47. See Lévi-Strauss (1967 [1958]). See also Mauss (1967 [1925]).
48. Irigaray 1985b.

49. Rubin 1990 [1976]: 75.
50. Ibid.: 80.
51. Presumably customers would like to select for "appropriate" gender as well as sex. The human engineers who discover how to make boys more "masculine" and girls more "feminine" will become wealthy indeed.
52. Rothschild 2000.
53. Rubin 1990 [1976]: 81–84.
54. Irigaray 1985b: 196–197.
55. Ibid.: 173. Irigaray uses the appellation "hom(m)o-sexual" to differentiate what we might call the homosocial masculine from the practices of male homosexuality that, as she points out, are forbidden (172).
56. The phallic kinship discourse of which the "male breadwinner" is emblematic is still alive and ideologically dominant today (Hochschield 1989), despite its prominent challenge by middle class feminists since the 1960s (e.g., Friedan 1983 [1963]), and despite the overwhelming majority of women now in the paid work force. The innumerable grueling realities of wage labor, however, are nothing to be glorified.
57. Lewin 1993.
58. E.g., de Lauretis (1992).

Chapter 6: Transforming the Means of Reproduction

1. Ferguson 1989: 286.
2. E.g., Evans 1978; Feinberg 1996; Grahn 1984.
3. Eskenazi et al. 1989.
4. Moraga 1997: 27.
5. Mamo 2002.
6. Rowland 1983, 1985.
7. Sullivan 1996.
8. Mamo 2002: 313.
9. Traiman 1998.
10. Rainbow Flag Health Services 2002.
11. TSBC 2002b.
12. Pies and Hornstein 1988.
13. Gartrell et al. 368.
14. See Nachtigall (1993) for a good discussion of the possible conflict of interest between parents and children in anonymous-donor AI.
15. Ibid.: 272–81.
16. This psychological legacy is not the same for adopted children all over the world. See Wegar (1997) for an exploration of how adoption discourses affect the differential valuation of children in Europe and the United States.
17. Rowland 1985.
18. Vanfraussen et al. 2001.

19. Ibid.
20. ABC 1998.
21. Ibid.
22. This particular list is from 1997, but similar ads are posted today.
23. Conception Connection 2002.
24. Weston 1998 [1995].
25. The widely unquestioned category of "high risk groups" is yet another way that language is used to reinforce oppression. As queer theorist Ellis Hanson (1991: 325) points out, this terminology transforms those hardest hit by AIDS into criminals. For even if AIDS were to have originated among Africans, African-Americans, or gay men, which as far as we know, it did not, these groups could hardly be claimed to be its source.

    The conflation of those hardest hit by the disease with the disease itself has fed a violent and widely played-out process of blaming the victim. In the United States, gay men have been the most publicized victims of this ideological sleight of hand, which portrays them in the media, and in the worlds of science, medicine, and religion, as AIDS personified.
26. The Sperm Bank of California 2002b.
27. These denotations are from Mamo (2002: 324–25).
28. Fenway Community Health 2002.
29. E.g., Brewaeys et al. 1993; Leiblum et al. 1995; Wendland et al. 1996. As noted earlier, the empirical evidence is scant, but growing. I am basing these conclusions on data drawn from research conducted in the United States, England, Belgium, and the Netherlands. While the legal and cultural status of lesbian AI is not identical in these countries, enough similarity exists to make the data meaningful.
30. Wendland et al. 1996.
31. Ibid.
32. Brewaeys et al. 1995.
33. Brewaeys et al. 1993.
34. Weston 1991: 171
35. E.g., European Parliament 1990; IHHS 1995; McCarrick 1996; Raymond 1993.
36. E.g., Kochler 1996; Rowland 1985.
37. E.g., Daniels 1995.
38. Brewaeys 2001.
39. Haimes 1998; 72, n.12.
40. Lui et al. 1995.
41. Daniels 1998: 93. See Stephenson and Wagner (1991) for a discussion of the many ways the practice of AI can be organized, as it is across Europe.
42. Early twentieth-century Italian anarchist Antonio Gramsci developed a theory of ideological hegemony that "takes Marx (the ruling ideas of every epoch are the ideas of the ruling class idea) one step further: The workers come to view themselves in the terms that the ruling class gives them. To the extent that subordinate

classes accept the ideas of the ruling class, the ideas are hegemonic" (Wehr 2002). Gramscian hegemony has been extended to include any powerful group's ability to impose its definitions of reality on those they dominate. The term "hegemony" also implies the ability, indeed the necessity, of those who are dominated to form their own definitions of reality, including their own oppression.

43. For good discussions of the construction of lesbians, lesbianism, and homosexuality as "unnatural" see Terry (1997); Terry and Urla (1995); Gibson (1997); and Foucault (1990 [1976]).

44. E.g., Alpert 1988; Miller 1992; Mohler and Frazer 2002; Noble 1987.

45. Pies 1989.

46. Ettelbrick 1997; Polikoff 1987; Robson 1998.

47. Martin 1993: 330–33.

48. Graff 1996.

49. Duggan 1997.

50. E.g. Sullivan 1997.

51. Gartrell et al. 2000: 546.

52. Gunning 1997.

53. E.g., Martin 1993. I put the "innocence" described above in quotation marks because such contexts are never really innocent of the heteronormativity that pervades kinship discourse. Assumptions about the proper place of women, men, children, sex, family, and kinship come to the fore when the presence of children rattles those chains of signification that hang so heavily on sex-gender-kinship nonconformists' necks.

54. JoAnn Loulan, personal communication 1995.

55. Gartrell 2000: 367.

56. E.g., Stack 1974; Rapp 1982.

57. Weston 1991.

58. Ibid.

59. For fascinating accounts of how this boundary work is micro-negotiated, see Weston (1991) and Lewin (1993).

60. Gartrell et al. 2000: 546.

61. Weston 1991.

62. Stacey 1996.

63. Martin 1993.

64. Stacey 1996; Stacey and Biblarz 2001; Stacey and Davenport 2002.

65. Sullivan 1996.

66. Ibid.

67. Carrington 1999: 15.

68. Ibid.

69. Ibid.: 216.

70. Ibid.: 215.

71. Ibid.

Chapter 7: Conclusions

1. West 1991 [1988]: 223.
2. Equitable estoppel is a legal doctrine that can be summarized as follows. When somebody has taken an action or made an assertion, with the intention of causing a second person to rely on the action or assertion, and that second person has in fact relied on it to their detriment, the first person will be not be permitted to take a position in court contrary to the original action or assertion. That first person loses a right that they would have had, because the court decides that it would be unfair to the second person to allow them to assert their right under those circumstances. So a sperm donor who relinquished paternal rights, and was chosen as the sperm donor for that reason, could be equitably estopped to assert his right to paternity in court.
3. Harlow 1996.
4. Harvard Law School 1990: 147.
5. While I am loathe to analogize between sexuality and race, the legalization of interracial marriage seems relevant here, since it expanded the meaning of marriage. *Loving* vs. *Virginia*, the Supreme Court's abolition of anti-miscegenation laws in 1968, did not reflect a national consensus, but rather implemented (progressive) social policy with the coercive force of law behind it. In 1968, most people (72% according to a Gallup poll) did not like the Supreme Court decision, which protected a tiny sexual/racial/kinship minority from a vast majority. As Sullivan points out (1997: xxi), today a significantly smaller majority (58%) oppose same-sex marriage, although majorities support protection of gays from discrimination in housing (84%) and employment (80%), as well as inheritance rights (61% to 29%), and a plurality support social security benefits for same-sex spouses (48% to 43%).
6. Rosenbloom 1996.
7. E.g., Arnup and Boyd 1995; Robsan 1992.
8. National Center for Lesbian Rights 1991–1992.
9. Gavigan 1995.
10. Whether lesbians are in fact more civilized than other couples when they break up is of course a matter for speculation given the absence of data.
11. For a lucid and provocative discussion of lesbian moms' behavior post-breakup, see Shulman (2000).
12. Millbank 1996.
13. Beardsley 2002.
14. This generative and sustained feminist activism in family law explains, in large part, why the bulk of my concluding discussion is about legal issues.
15. Minow 1991: 272.
16. Ibid.: 282.
17. Harvard Law School 1991: 1651.
18. Minow 1991: 276–77.

19. Harvard Law School 1991: 1641.
20. Ibid.: 1653.
21. Ibid.: 1641.
22. Henry 1993.
23. Kendall and Haaland 1996: 41.
24. Schultz 1990: 297.
25. Pies 1985; Kendall and Haaland 1996.
26. E.g., Gilligan 1982; Jack and Jack 1989; Thorne 1993.
27. Jack and Jack 1989.
28. Collins 1990.
29. Jack and Jack 1989.
30. These definitions are shaped by the fact that the United States was founded on historical and legally enforced notions that an enslaved black person was only three-fifths of a human being, that one had to own property and be male to vote, and that women and children were owned and controlled by their fathers and husbands, as well as other constitutional edicts that form the bases for legal and cultural precedents to this day.
31. Williams 1991.
32. E.g., Pateman 1988.
33. Testy 1995.
34. Ibid.: 219.
35. Woodhouse 1993: 1786, cf. 150.
36. Fineman 1995.
37. Polikoff 1996.
38. Gender-neutral laws are more likely to be enacted than those that favor mothers.
39. Polikoff 1990.
40. Polikoff 1996: 375.
41. Ibid.: 393–394.
42. E.g., Post 1997; Ettelbrick 1997.
43. MacKinnon 1991 [1983]: 195.
44. This emphasis on sexual sameness was as ideologically fraught as the difference-based anatomies of the Victorians (and was equally dedicated to strengthening heteropatriarchal marriage). By framing and marketing their therapeutic interventions as "repairing the conjugal bed" (Irvine 1990: 90), these sexologists defended the institution of marriage and deflected attention from the sexism and social inequality that contribute to "sexual dysfunction" in U.S. marriages (Ibid.: 86–94). This shift to viewing men's and women's bodies as essentially similar was pioneered by Masters and Johnson who "discovered" (invented) the four-stage, gender-neutral, human sexual response cycle (1966).
45. Koontz 1997.
46. Sociologist Kathleen Gerson's (1993) extensive study of "men's changing commitments to family and work" found that 13 percent of fathers report that they "have

or planned to become equal or primary caretakers" (Ibid.: 13). As Gerson notes, this is a significant increase from thirty years ago, but does not change the basic dimensions of the gendered division of "parenting" labor.

47. Cuthbert et al. 2002.

48. For a discussion of these issues, see Chesler (1987) and Women's Rights Network (2002).

49. Fineman 1995: 163.

50. Slaughter 1995: 2161.

51. Gilligan 1982.

52. Wittig 1990 [1980].

53. This phrase is adopted from Donna Haraway, who wrote that her "Cyborg Manifesto" ". . . is an argument for pleasure in the confusion of boundaries and for responsibility in their construction" (1991: 150).

54. Fineman 1995: 2158.

55. One in five U.S. children is born poor, and one in three will be poor at some point before he or she is eighteen (Children's Defense Fund 2001).

56. U.S. Census Bureau 1997. In 1997, just over half (54%) of "custodial parents" (divorced or never-married moms) below the poverty level received any of their court-ordered child support at all. Two-thirds of all "custodial parents" received any of their court-ordered child support. Only a quarter (24%) of custodial parents below the poverty line received all court-ordered child support payments. For custodial parents above the poverty line, 40.9 percent received all their court-ordered payments. Of course, the latter figures in both statements include recipients above and below the poverty line, so the difference between the two groups is even larger than these numbers imply. Still, it is an abysmal performance, especially for wealthy fathers whose own standard of living has generally gone up after divorce (Coontz 1997: 138). It also bears noting that these numbers exclude fathers who are incarcerated or otherwise "institutionalized," which is a significant percentage of all U.S. fathers.

57. Woodhouse 1993: 1752.

58. Woodhouse 1993: 1766.

59. Shanley 2001: 125–26.

60. Ibid.: 139.

61. Woodhouse 1993: 1785.

62. Shanley 2001: 125–126.

63. Woodhouse 2001.

64. This was pointed out by Professor Michael Grodin in a small group session on children's rights in the Short Course in Health and Human Rights, Harvard School of Public Health, 19 June 2002.

65. Vagelatos 1995: 140.

66. West 1991 [1988]: 233.

67. Rafkin 1990.

68. Blumenfeld 1992.

69. Ross 1996.
70. For more on "street theory" and its relationship to "straight theory" see Weston (1998).
71. Allison 1977.
72. As I have discussed earlier, lesbians engaged in custody battles also draw on whatever available cultural and discursive resources they believe will help them win. Such arguments may do little to further the lesbian *nomos,* and may even detract from it.
73. Admittedly, this viewpoint implies that biological fathers need have no financial responsibilities toward their offspring if a social relationship has not been developed. Obviously this requires dignified welfare-state guarantees for mothers and children, so that they will not be dependent on the generosity of wealthy or wealthier men.
74. Rothman 1989.
75. Bob Defandorf coined the term "immasculate conception" (personal conversation, 1997).

Appendix A: Methodology, Sources, and Citations

1. I do not claim, however, to "triangulate" among these sources, since that would be to overstate the level of certainty that is often possible in the rapidly changing area of lesbian AI. At one time I felt "triangulation" closely described my methodology. That was before being persuaded by numerous arguments that the term is too fundamentally problematic to apply to my work, and possibly to any social science research. For a good overview of this argument, please see Massey (1999).
2. Vizenor 1990: 412.
3. Foucault 1990 [1976]: 96.
4. Epistemology is a term from philosophy that refers to the study of how it is we know what we know. Because epistemologies have to do with our perceptions of what reality is, they are the basis of important relationships between selves and others, between our bodies and the world, between language and technologies, and among all kinds of social and political structures and institutions. Epistemologies are so deeply embedded in the fabric of our experiences that we take them to be natural. Thus, alternative epistemologies can productively destabilize perception.
5. Pfohl 1992: 174–77.
6. This is important to ask since not all inseminations result in conception and birth.

Appendix B: Definitions

1. O'Neill 1985: 49.
2. For a good discussion of earlier second-wave debates, see Ferguson (1989), chapter 9. For a fascinating discussion of more contemporary debates, including their application to legal issues, see Robson (1998), chapter 4.
3. Unfortunately, potential inseminees and their partners cannot always trust that the fresh sperm they receive is actually that of a stranger. While rare, there have been

cases such as that of Dr. Cecil B. Jacobson, an Alexandria, Virginia, infertility specialist convicted in 1992 of using his own sperm to impregnate at least nine patients (Ginsburg 1997: cf. note 823).

4. Petchesky 1987.
5. E.g., Noble 1987.
6. E.g., Weston 1991.
7. E.g., Santa Cruz Women's Health Collective 1979.
8. E.g., Klein 1984.
9. E.g., Barlet and Penney 1994.
10. Annas 1980.
11. Daniels 1998.
12. Firestone 2000: 55–56.
13. Huxley 1998 [1932]. In Huxley's dystopia, people are bioengineered for maximum efficiency and profitability, and lulled into life-long complacency with propaganda, sex, and drugs.
14. Rothman 1989.
15. American Society for Reproductive Medicine 2001b.
16. Doane and Hodges 1987: 6. To learn more about the diverse types of feminism, I recommend starting with a good feminist reference work (e.g., Kramarae and Spender 2000, or Mankiller et al. 1998). These give the reader the benefit of a brief introduction written by experts in each area of feminism, rather than the perspective of a single author, no matter how brilliant. Also, each entry will have carefully selected citations for further reading.
17. Aptheker's definition of feminism was later published in "Memories of the Free Speech Movement" (Aptheker 1995).
18. Sociologist Andrea Walsh first shared this quotation with me. Handout in author's personal collection.
19. Rebecca West, circa 1913. Quoted in Briggs 1996: 137.
20. For more on lesbian choices not necessarily being feminist choices, see Calhoun (1996).

Works Cited

ABC. 1998. "Faceless, Nameless Fathers: Donor Offspring Search for Clues about their Dads." New York: ABC News.

Abma, J., A. Chandra, W. Mosher, L. Peterson, and I. Piccinino. 1997. "Fertility, Family Planning, and Women's Health: New Data from the 1995 National Survey of Family Growth." National Center for Health Statistics. *Vital Health Stat* 23, no. 19.

Alexander, M. Jacqui. 1991. "Redrafting Morality: The Postcolonial State and the Sexual Offenses Bill of Trinidad and Tobago." In *Third World Women and the Politics of Feminism,* edited by A.R. Chandra Talpade Mohanty and Lourdes Torres, 133–52. Bloomington and Indianapolis: Indiana University Press.

Allen, Paula Gunn. 1986. *The Sacred Hoop: Recovering the Feminine in American Indian Traditions.* Boston: Beacon Press.

Allison, Dorothy. 1977. "Keynote Speech." San Francisco: National Center for Lesbian Rights.

Alpert, Harriet. 1988. *We Are Everywhere: Writings by and About Lesbian Parents.* Freedom, Calif.: The Crossing Press.

American Academy of Pediatrics, Committee on Psychosocial Aspects of Child and Family Health. 2002. "Policy Statement: Coparent or Second-Parent Adoption by Same-Sex Parents." *Pediatrics* 109, no. 3: 339–40.

American Academy of Pediatrics, Ellen C. Perrin, MD, and the Committee on Psychosocial Aspects of Child and Family Health. 2002. "Technical Report: Coparent or Second-Parent Adoption by Same-Sex Parents." *Pediatrics* 109, no. 2: 341–44.

American Civil Liberties Union, Lesbian and Gay Rights Freedom Network. "'Crime' and Punishment in America: State-by-State Breakdown of Sodomy Laws." <http://www.aclu.org/issues/gay/sodomy.html>, accessed 28 June 2002.

American Society for Reproductive Medicine (The American Fertility Society). 1990.

"Revised Minimum Standards for In Vitro Fertilization, Gamete Intrafallopian Transfer, and Related Procedures." *Fertility and Sterility* 53.

———. 1996a. "State Infertility Insurance Laws." <http://www.asrm.com>, accessed 7/18/1997.

———, Board of Directors, 1996b. "Guidelines for the Provision of Infertility Services." Edited by ASRM Practice Committee. Birmingham, Ala.: ASRM.

———. 1996–1997. "Fact Sheet: Intracytoplasmic Sperm Injection (ICSI)." Birmingham, Ala.: ASRM.

———. 1997. "Guidelines for Gamete and Embryo Donation: A Practice Committee Report, Guidelines and Minimum Standards." <http://asrm.org/Media/Practice/gamete.html>, accessed 27 June 2002.

———, Ethics Committee. 2001a. "Ethics Committee Report: Preconception Gender Selection for Nonmedical Reasons." *Fertility and Sterility* 75, no. 5: 861–64.

———. 2001b. "State Infertility Insurance Laws." <http://www.asrm.org/Patients/insur.html>, accessed 5 June 2002. Dated June 2001.

Andrews, Lori. 1999. *The Clone Age: Adventures in the New World of Reproductive Technology.* New York: Henry Holt and Company.

Annas, George. 1980. "Fathers Anonymous: Beyond the Best Interests of the Sperm Donor." *Family Law Quarterly* 14: 1–13.

Anzaldùa, Gloria. 1990a. *Making Face, Making Soul = Haciendo Caras: Creative and Critical Perspectives by Women of Color.* San Francisco: Aunt Lute Foundation Books.

———. 1990b. "La conciencia de la mestiza: Towards a New Consciousness." In *Making Face, Making Soul = Haciendo Caras: Creative and Critical Perspectives by Women of Color,* edited by Gloria Anzaldùa, 377–89. San Francisco: Aunt Lute Foundation Books.

Aptheker, Bettina. 1995. "Memories of FSM [Free Speech Movement]." In *Takin' It to the Streets,* edited by A. Bloom and N. Breines. New York: Oxford University Press.

Arms, Suzanne. 1975. *Immaculate Deception: A New Look at Women and Childbirth.* New York: Bantam.

Arnup, Katherine, and Susan Boyd. 1995. "Familial Disputes? Sperm Donors, Lesbian Mothers, and Legal Parenthood." In *Legal Inversions: Lesbians, Gay Men, and the Politics of Law,* edited by Didi Herman, and Carl Stychin, 77–1001. Philadelphia: Temple University Press.

Augustin, Nathalie A. 1997. "Learnfare and Black Motherhood: The Social Construction of Deviance." In *Critical Race Feminism: A Reader,* edited by A.K. Wing, 144–50. New York and London: New York University Press.

Badgett, L. 1995. "The Wage Effects of Sexual Orientation Discrimination." *Industrial and Labor Relations Review* 48, no. 4: 726–39.

Baldauf, Scott. 1997. "How Texas Wrestles with Gay Adoptions." *The Christian Science Monitor* 3 December.

Baran, Annette, and Reuben Pannor. 1989. *Lethal Secrets: The Shocking Consequences and Unsolved Problems of Artificial Insemination.* New York: Warner Books.

Barlet, E.M., and L.L. Penney. 1994. "Therapeutic Donor Insemination: Fresh Versus Frozen." *Missouri Med* 91: 85–88.

Bartlett, Katherine T. 1984. "Rethinking Parenthood as an Exclusive Status: The Need for Legal Alternatives When the Promise of the Nuclear Family Has Failed." *Virginia Law Review* 70: 879–963.

——. 1990. "Feminist Legal Methods." *Harvard Law Review* 103: 830–65.

Bartlett, Katherine T., and Rosanne Kennedy. 1991. *Feminist Legal Theory: Readings in Law and Gender.* Boulder, San Francisco, and Oxford: Westview Press.

Baudrillard, Jean. 1988. *Jean Baudrillard: Selected Writings.* Edited and Introduced by Mark Poster. Translated by Paul, Foss, Paul Patton, and Philip Beitchman (selection translators). Stanford: Stanford University Press.

Beauvoir, Simone de. 1993 [1953]. *The Second Sex.* New York: Alfred A. Knopf: Distributed by Random House.

Belsey, Catherine. 1980. *Critical Practice.* London: Methuen and Company Ltd.

Beardsley, Elisabeth J. 2002. "Landmark Ruling Forces Lesbian to Pay Support." *Boston Globe,* Thursday, 18 July 2002.

Benkov, Laura. 1994. *Reinventing the Family: Lesbian and Gay Parents.* New York: Crown Trade Paperbacks.

Bersani, Leo. 1988. "Is the Rectum a Grave?" In *AIDS: Cultural Analysis, Cultural Activism,* edited by D. Crimp. Cambridge and London: MIT Press.

Beuren, Geraldine Van. 1995. "The International Protection of Family Members' Rights as the 21st Century Approaches." *Human Rights Quarterly* 17: 732–765.

Blank, Robert H. 1998. "Regulation of Donor Insemination." In *Donor Insemination: International Social Science Perspectives,* edited by Ken Daniels and Erica Haimes, 131–50. Cambridge, England: University of Cambridge Press.

Blankenhorn, David. 1995. *Fatherless America: Confronting Our Most Urgent Social Problem.* New York: Basic Books.

Blumenfeld, Warren J. 1992. *Homophobia: How We All Pay the Price.* Boston: Beacon Press.

Boggis, Terry. 2001. "Affording Our Families: Class Issues in Family Formation." In *Queer Families, Queer Politics,* edited by Mary Bernstein and Renate Reimann, 175–81. New York: Routledge.

Boston Women's Health Book Collective. 1992. *The New Our Bodies, Ourselves: A Book by and for Women: Updated and Expanded for the '90s.* New York: Simon & Schuster.

Brewaeys, Anne. 2001. "Review: Parent-Child Relationships and Child Development in Donor Insemination Families." *Human Reproduction Update* 7, no. 1: 38–46.

Brewaeys, Anne, I. Ponjaert-Kristoffersen, A.C. Van Steirteghem, and P. Devroey. 1993. "Children from Anonymous Donors: An Inquiry into Homosexual and Heterosexual Parents' Attitudes." *Journal of Psychosomatic Obstetrics and Gynaecology* 14: 23–35.

Brewaeys, Anne, P. Devroey, F.M. Helmerhorst, E.V. Van Hall, and I. Ponjaert. 1995. "Lesbian Mothers Who Conceived after Donor Insemination: A Follow-up Study." *Journal of Human Reproduction* 10: 2731–35.

Bridges, Amy, and Heidi Hartmann. 1981. "The Unhappy Marriage of Marxism and

Feminism: Towards a More Progressive Union." In *Women and Revolution: A Discussion of the Unhappy Marriage of Marxism and Feminism,* edited by L. Sargent, 1–41. Boston: South End Press.

Briggs, Mary, ed. 1996. *Women's Words: The Columbia Book of Quotations by Women.* New York: Columbia University Press.

Bruhl, Elise. 2000/2001. "Motherhood and Contract: Always Crashing in the Same Car." *Buffalo Women's Law Journal* 9: 191–224.

Buchwald, Emilie, Pamela R. Fletcher, and Martha Roth, eds. *Transforming a Rape Culture.* Minneapolis: Milkweed Editions.

Burnham, Margaret. 1993 [1987]. "An Impossible Marriage: Slave Law and Family Law." In *Family Matters: Readings on Family Lives and the Law,* edited by M. Minow, 142–56. New York: The New Press.

Calhoun, C. 1996. "Must Lesbian Choices Be Feminist Choices?" *Journal of Homosexuality* 32: 7–20.

California Cryobank, Inc. 1998. "Racial Identification System." Los Angeles: California Cryobank, Inc.

———. 2002. "Andrology Services." <http://www1.cryobank.com/andro.cfm?page=3&sub=6>, accessed 15 August 2002.

———. 2003. "Semen Specimen Quality Assurance System." <http://www.cryobank.com/racial.cfm?page=3&sub=4>, accessed 10 January 2003.

———. 2003a. "The Keirsey Temperament Sorter." <http://www.cryobank.com/keirsey.cfm>, accessed 13 June 2003.

———. 2003b. "Donor Profiles." <http://www.cryobank.com/profile.cfm>, accessed 13 June 2003.

———. 2003c. "Power Search." <http://www.cryobank.com/search/index.cfm?toppage=4>, accessed 16 June 2003.

Cambridge Documentary Films. 2002. *Rape Is . . .* <http://www.cambridgedocumentaryfilms.org/rapeis-info.html>, accessed 18 August 2002.

Carby, Hazel V. 1987. *Reconstructing Womanhood: The Emergence of the Afro-American Woman Novelist.* New York: Oxford University Press.

Carrington, Christopher. 1999. *No Place Like Home: Relationships and Family Life among Lesbians and Gay Men.* Chicago and London: University of Chicago Press.

Chambers, David L. 1996. "What If? The Legal Consequences of Marriage and the Legal Needs of Lesbian and Gay Male Couples." *Michigan Law Review* 95: 447–91.

Chambers-Schiller, Lee Virginia. 1984. *Liberty, A Better Husband: Single Women in America: The Generations of 1780–1840.* New Haven and London: Yale University Press.

Chesler, Phyllis. 1987. *Mothers on Trial: The Battle for Children and Custody.* Seattle: The Seal Press.

Children's Defense Fund. 2001. "The State of America's Children Yearbook 2001: twenty-five Key Facts about American Children." <http://www.childrensdefense.org/keyfacts.htm>, accessed 31 August 2002.

Cixous, Hélène. 1976 [1975]. "The Laugh of the Medusa." Translated by Keith Cohen and Paula Cohen. *Signs* 1: 875–93.

Clarke, Adele E., and Virginia L. Olesen, eds. 1999. *Revisioning Women, Health, and Healing: Feminist, Cultural, and Technoscience Perspectives.* New York: Routledge.

Cleaver, Kathleen Neal. 1997. "Racism, Civil Rights, and Feminism." In *Critical Race Feminism, Critical America,* edited by A.K. Wing, 35–43. New York and London: New York University Press.

Colen, Shellee. 1989. "Just a Little Respect": West Indian Domestic Workers in New York City." Chap. 9 In *Muchachas No More: Household Workers in Latin America and the Caribbean,* edited by Elsa M. Chaney and Mary Garcia Castro, 171-194. Philadelphia: Temple University Press.

Colker, Ruth. 1996. "Pregnant Men Revisited or Sperm Is Cheap, Eggs Are Not." *Hastings Law Journal* 47 (April) 1063–80.

Collins, Patricia Hill. 1990. *Black Feminist Thought: Knowledge, Consciousness, and the Politics of Empowerment.* New York: Unwin Hyman.

Conception Connection. 2002. "Registry and Counseling Service." <http://www.alternativefamilies.org/conception.html>, accessed 21 June 2002.

Conrad, Peter. 1992. "Medicalization and Social Control." *Annual Review of Sociology* 18: 209–32.

Conrad, Peter, and Rochelle Kern. 1990. *The Sociology of Health and Illness: Critical Perspectives.* Third Edition. New York: St. Martin's Press.

Convention on the Rights of the Child, The. Unanimously adopted by the United Nations General Assembly on 20 November 1989, and entered into force in September 1990.

Coontz, Stephanie. 1997. *The Way We Really Are: Coming to Terms with America's Changing Families.* New York: Basic Books/Harper Collins.

Cooper, Davina, and Didi Herman. 1995. "Getting 'The Family Right': Legislating Heterosexuality in Britain, 1986–91." In *Legal Inversions: Lesbians, Gay Men, and the Politics of Law,* edited by Didi Herman and Carl Stychin, 162–79. Philadelphia: Temple University Press.

Corea, Gena. 1985. *The Mother Machine: Reproductive Technology from Artificial Insemination to Artificial Wombs.* New York: Harper and Row.

Crimmins, Barry. 1988. "Strange Bedfellows: Comedy and Politics," edited by various artists. Hollywood, California: A&M Records. Sound recording.

Curie-Cohen, M. 1979. "Current Practice of Artificial Insemination by Donor in the United States." *New England Journal of Medicine* 300: 585–90.

Cuthbert, C., K. Slote, M.G. Driggers, C.J. Mesh, L. Bancroft, and J. Silverman. 2002. *Battered Mothers Speak Out: A Human Rights Report on Domestic Violence and Child Custody in the Massachusetts Family Courts.* Wellesley, Mass.: Wellesley Centers for Women.

Daly, Mary. 1984. *Pure Lust: Elemental Feminist Philosophy.* Boston: Beacon Press.

Daniels, Ken. 1995. "Information Sharing in AI: A Conflict of Needs and Rights." *Cambridge Quarterly of Healthcare Ethics* 4: 217–24.

————. 1998. "The Semen Providers." In *Donor Insemination: International Social Science Perspectives,* edited by Ken Daniels and Erica Haimes, 76–104. Cambridge: University of Cambridge Press.

Daniels, Ken, and Erica Haimes. 1998. *Donor Insemination: International Social Science Perspectives.* Cambridge: University of Cambridge Press.

Davis, Angela Y. 1981. *Women, Race and Class.* New York: Vintage Books.

De Lauretis, Teresa, ed. 1992. "The Phallus Issue." *Differences: A Journal of Feminist Cultural Studies* 4, no. 1.

Delaney, Elizabeth A. 1991. "Statutory Protection of the Other Mother: Legally Recognizing the Relationship between the Nonbiological Lesbian Parent and Her Child." *Hastings Law Journal* 43: 177–216.

Derrida, Jacques. 1976. *Of Grammatology.* Translated by Gayatri Chakravorti Spivak. Baltimore and London: The Johns Hopkins University Press.

DiMarzo, S.J., J. Huang, J.F. Kennedy, B. Villanueva, S.A. Hebert, and P.E. Young. 1990. "Pregnancy Rates with Fresh Versus Computer-Controlled Cryopreserved Semen for Artificial Insemination by Donor in a Private Practice Setting." *American Journal of Obstetrics and Gynecology* 162: 1483–88.

Doane, Janice, and Devon Hodges. 1987. *Nostalgia and Sexual Difference: The Resistance to Contemporary Feminism.* New York and London: Methuen.

Doyal, Lesley. 1995. *What Makes Women Sick: Gender and the Political Economy of Health.* New Jersey: Rutgers University Press.

Duberman, Martin B., Martha Vicinus, and George Chauncey. 1991. *Hidden from History: Reclaiming the Gay and Lesbian Past.* London: Penguin.

Duggan, Kathy. 1997. "I Earned This Divorce." In *Same-Sex Marriage: Pro and Con: A Reader,* edited by Andrew Sullivan, 300–302. New York: Vintage.

Duka, Walter E., and Alan H. DeCherney. 1996. *From the Beginning: A History of the American Fertility Society 1944–1994.* Birmingham, Ala.: American Society for Reproductive Medicine.

Durkheim, Emile. 1990 [1912]. *The Elementary Forms of the Religious Life, a Study in Religious Sociology.* Translated by Joseph W. Swain. New York: The Free Press.

Dyer, Richard. 1990 [1985]. "Coming to Terms." In *Out There: Marginalization and Contemporary Culture,* edited by R. Ferguson, Martha Gever, Trinh T. Minh-ha, and Cornel West, 289–98. New York, Cambridge and London: The New Museum of Contemporary Art and the MIT Press.

Eaton, Mary. 1995. "Homosexual Unmodified: Speculations on Law's Discourse, Race, and the Construction of Sexual Identity." In *Legal Inversions: Lesbians, Gay Men, and the Politics of Law,* edited by Didi Herman and Carl Stychin, 46–73. Philadelphia: Temple University Press.

Ehrenreich, Barbara, 1983. *The Hearts of Men: American Dreams and the Flight from Commitment.* New York: Anchor Books/Doubleday.

Ehrenreich, Barbara, and Deirdre English. 1973. *Complaints and Disorders: The Sexual Politics of Sickness.* Old Westbury, N.Y.: The Feminist Press.

Eisenstein, Zillah. 1998. *Global Obscenities: Patriarchy, Capitalism, and the Lure of Cyberfantasy.* New York: New York University Press.

Engels, Frederick. 1963 [1884]. *The Origin of the Family, Private Property, and the State. In the Light of the Research.* New York: International Publishers.

Englert, Y. 1994. "Artificial Insemination of Single Women and Lesbian Women with Donor Semen." *Human Reproduction* 9: 1969–71.

Ernulf, K.E., S.M. Innala, and F.L. Whitam. 1989. "Biological Explanation, Psychological Explanation, and Tolerance of Homosexuals: A Cross-National Analysis of Beliefs and Attitudes." *Psychology of Reproduction* 65 (3 Part 1): 1003–10.

Eskenazi, B., C. Pies, A. Newsletter, C. Shepard, and K. Pearson. 1989. "HIV Serology in Artificially Inseminated Lesbians." *Journal of Acquired Immune Deficiency Syndrome* 2, no. 2: 187–93.

Ettelbrick, Paula. 1997. "Since When Is Marriage a Path to Liberation?" In *Same-Sex Marriage: Pro and Con: A Reader,* edited by Andrew Sullivan, 118–24. New York: Vintage.

European Parliament, Committee on Legal Affairs, Citizens Rights. 1990. *Ethical and Legal Problems of Genetic Engineering and Human Artificial Insemination.* Luxembourg: Office for Official Publications of the European Communities; Lanham.

Evans, Arthur. 1978. *Witchcraft and the Gay Counterculture: A Radical View of Western Civilization and Some of the People It Has Tried to Destroy.* Boston: Fag Rag Books.

Faderman, Lillian. 1981. *Surpassing the Love of Men: Romantic Friendship and Love between Women from the Renaissance to the Present.* New York: William Morrow.

Fairfax Cryobank. 2002. "Home Page." <http://www.fairfaxcryobank.com>, accessed 15 August 2002.

———. 2003. "Fairfax Cryobank Information Center." <http://www.fairfaxcryobank .com/cryo/shoppingcart/search.cfm>, accessed 16 June 2003.

Fanon, Frantz. 1961. *The Wretched of the Earth.* Translated by Constance Farrington. Paris, France: Grove Press.

Farquhar, Dion. 1996. *The Other Machine: Discourse and Reproductive Technologies.* New York and London: Routledge.

———. 1999. "Gamete Traffic/Pedestrian Crossing." In *Playing Dolly: Technocultural Formations, Fantasies, and Fictions of Assisted Reproduction,* edited by E. Ann Kaplan and Susan Squier, 17–36. New Brunswick, N.J.: Rutgers University Press.

Fenway Community Health. 2002. "Family and Parenting Services: Alternative Insemination." <http://www.fenwayhealth.org/services/alternative/alternat.htm>, accessed 17 August 2002.

Ferguson, Anne. 1989. *Blood at the Root: Motherhood, Sexuality and Male Dominance.* London: Pandora.

Field, Martha A. 1990. *Surrogate Motherhood: The Legal and Human Issues.* Cambridge and London: Harvard University Press.

Feinberg, Leslie. 1996. *Transgender Warriors: Making History from Joan of Arc to RuPaul.* Boston: Beacon Press.

Fineman, Martha Albertson. 1995. *The Neutered Mother, the Sexual Family, and Other Twentieth Century Tragedies*. New York and London: Routledge.

Fineman, Martha Albertson, and Nancy Sweet Thomadsen, eds. 1991. *At the Boundaries of the Law: Feminism and Legal Theory*. New York and London: Routledge.

Fineman, Martha Albertson, and Isabel Karpin. 1995. *Mothers in Law: Feminist Theory and the Legal Regulation of Motherhood*. New York: Columbia University Press.

Firestone, Jenifer. 2000. "The State of the State of Queer Parenting." In *Home Fronts: Controversies in Nontraditional Parenting*, edited by Jess Wells, 25–60. Los Angeles and New York: Alyson Books.

Foucault, Michel. 1990 [1976]. *The History of Sexuality*, volume 1: *An Introduction*. Translated by Robert Hurley. New York: Vintage Books.

Franklin, Sarah. 1992. "Making Representations: The Parliamentary Debate on the Human Fertilisation and Embryology Act." In *Technologies of Procreation: Kinship in the Age of Assisted Conception*, edited by Jeanette Edwards, 128. Manchester, England: Manchester University Press.

———. 1995. "Postmodern Procreation: A Cultural Account of Assisted Reproduction." In *Conceiving the New World Order: The Global Politics of Reproduction*, edited by Faye D. Ginsburg and Rayna Rapp, 323–45. Berkeley: University of California Press.

Friedan, Betty. 1983 [1963]. *The Feminine Mystique*. New York: Dell Publishing Co.

Fuss, Diana. 1989. *Essentially Speaking: Feminism, Nature & Difference*. New York: Routledge.

Gartrell, Nanette, Jean Hamilton, Amy Banks, Dee Mosbacher, Nancy Reed, C. Sparks, and Holly Bishop. 1996. "The National Lesbian Family Study 1: Interviews with Prospective Mothers." *American Journal of Orthopsychiatry* 66: 272–81.

Gartrell, Nanette, Amy Banks, Jean Hamilton, Nancy Reed, Holly Bishop, and Carla Rodas. 1999. "The National Lesbian Family Study 2: Interviews with Mothers and Toddlers." *American Journal of Orthopsychiatry* 69, no. 3: 362–69.

Gartrell, Nanette, Amy Banks, Nancy Reed, Jean Hamilton, Carla Rodas, and Amalia Deck. 2000. "The National Lesbian Family Study 3: Interviews with Mothers of Five-Year-Olds." *American Journal of Orthopsychiatry* 70, no. 4: 542–48.

Gavigan, Shelley A.M. 1995. "A Parent(ly) Knot: Can Heather Have Two Mommies?" In *Legal Inversions: Lesbians, Gay Men, and the Politics of Law*, edited by Didi Herman and Carl Stychin, 102–17. Philadelphia: Temple University Press.

Geertz, Clifford. 1983. *Local Knowledge: Further Essays in Interpretive Anthropology*. New York: Basic Books.

Genetics and IVF Institute. 2002. "MicroSort Sperm Separation." http://www. microsort .net, accessed 31 August 2002.

Gerson, Kathleen. 1993. *No Man's Land: Men's Changing Commitments to Family and Work*. New York: Basic Books.

Gibson, Margaret. 1997. "Clitoral Corruption: Body Metaphors and American Doctors' Constructions of Female Homosexuality, 1870–1900." In *Science and Homosexualities*, edited by Vernon Rosario, 108–32. New York and London: Routledge.

Gideonse, Ted. 1997. "The Sexual Blur: With Straights Falling for Gays, Lesbians Dating Men, and Gay Men in Love with Women, Is Anybody Anything Anymore? Just How Important *Is* Sexual Identity? *The Advocate,* 24 June 1997. <http://www.advocate.com/html/stories/820/820_blur736.asp>, accessed 17 July 2002.

Gilligan, Carol. 1982. *In a Different Voice: Psychological Theory and Women's Development.* Cambridge and London; Harvard University Press.

Gilman, Charlotte Perkins. (as Charlotte Perkins Stetson.) 1966 [1898]. *Women and Economics: A Study of the Economic Relation between Men and Women as a Factor in Social Evolution.* New York: Harper & Row.

Ginsburg, Karen. 1997. "Note: FDA Approved? A Critique of the Artificial Insemination Industry in the United States." *Michigan Journal of Law Reform* (Summer), 30 U. Mich. J.L. Ref. 823.

Goldman, Emma. 1970 [1917]. *The Traffic in Women and Other Essays on Feminism.* Ojai, California: Times Change Press.

Goldstein, Joseph, Anna Freud, and Albert J. Solnit. 1973. *Beyond the Best Interests of the Child.* New York: Free Press.

Gough, Kathleen. 1975. "The Origin of the Family." In *Toward an Anthropology of Women,* edited by Rayna [Rapp] Reiter, 67–70. New York: Monthly Review Press.

Graff, E.J. 1996. "Retying the Knot." In *Same-Sex Marriage: Pro and Con: A Reader,* edited by Andrew Sullivan, 134–38. New York: Vintage.

Grahn, Judy. 1984. *Another Mother Tongue: Gay Words, Gay Worlds.* Boston: Beacon Press.

Greil, Arthur L. 1990. *Not Yet Pregnant: Infertile Couples in Contemporary America.* New Brunswick and London: Rutgers University Press.

Gunning, Isabelle R. 1997. "A Story from Home: On Being a Black Lesbian Mother." In *Critical Race Feminism: A Reader,* edited by A.K. Wing, 159–62. New York and London: New York University Press.

Haimes, Erica. 1998. "The Making of 'the DI Child': Changing Representations of People Conceived through Donor Insemination." In *Donor Insemination: International Social Science Perspectives,* edited by Ken Daniels and Erica Haimes, 53–75. Cambridge; University of Cambridge Press.

Hanscombe, Gillian E., and Jackie Forster. 1982. *Rocking the Cradle. Lesbian Mothers: A Challenge in Family Living.* Boston: Alyson Publications.

Hansen, Karen V., and Irene J. Philipson, eds. 1990. *Women, Class, and the Feminist Imagination: A Socialist-Feminist Reader.* Philadelphia; Temple University Press.

Hanson, Ellis. 1991. "Undead." In *Inside/Out: Lesbian Theories, Gay Theories,* edited by D. Fuss, 321–40. New York and London: Routledge.

Haraway, Donna J. 1991. "A Cyborg Manifesto: Science, Technology, and Socialist-Feminism in the Late Twentieth Century." In *Simians, Cyborgs, and Women: The Reinvention of Nature.* New York and London: Routledge.

Haraway, Donna J. 1997. *Modest_Witness@Second_Millennium.FemaleMan©_Meets_OncoMouse*™: Feminism and Technoscience. New York: Routledge.

Harlow, Holly J. 1996. "Paternalism without Paternity: Discrimination against Single Women Seeking Artificial Insemination by Donor." *Southern California Review of Law and Women's Studies* 6: 173.

Hartouni, Valerie. 1997. *Cultural Conceptions: On Reproductive Technologies and the Remaking of Life.* Minneapolis: University of Minnesota Press.

Hartouni, Valerie. 1999. "A Study in Reproductive Technologies." In *Revisioning Women, Health and Healing: Feminist, Cultural, and Technoscience Perspectives,* edited by Adele E. Clarke and Virginia L. Olesen, 254–65. New York: Routledge.

Harvard Law School: Editors of the Harvard Law Review. 1990. *Sexual Orientation and the Law.* Cambridge and London: Harvard University Press.

———. "Looking for a Family Resemblance: The Limit of the Functional Approach to the Legal Definition of the Family." Harvard Law Review ??MS 358 Note 104: 1640–59.??

Henry, Vickie L. 1993. "A Tale of Three Women: A Survey of the Rights and Responsibilities of Unmarried Women Who Conceive by Alternative Insemination and a Model for Legislative Reform." *American Journal of Law & Medicine* 19: 285–310.

Hitchens, Donna J. 1985. "Legal Issues in Donor Insemination." In *Considering Parenthood: A Workbook for Lesbians,* edited by C. Pies, 215–26. San Francisco: Spinsters/Aunt Lute.

Hochschield, Arlie. 1989. *The Second Shift: Working Parents and the Revolution at Home.* New York: Viking Penguin.

Holmstrom, Nancy, ed. 2002. *The Socialist Feminist Project: A Contemporary Reader in Theory and Politics.* New York: The Monthly Review Press.

hooks, bell. 1984. *Feminist Theory: From Margin to Center.* Boston: South End Press.

Howard-Hassman, Rhoda E. 2001. "Gay Rights and the Right to a Family: Conflicts between Liberal and Illiberal Belief Systems." *Human Rights Quarterly* 23: 73–95.

Hubbard, Ruth. 1990. *The Politics of Women's Biology.* New Brunswick, N.J.: Rutgers University Press.

Hull, Gloria T., Barbara Smith, and Patricia Bell-Scott. 1982. *All the Women are White, All the Blacks are Men, But Some of Us Are Brave: Black Women's Studies.* Old Westbury, N.Y.: Feminist Press.

Human Rights Campaign Fund. 2003. "HRC FamilyNet: Legal Documents to Protect Your Family." <http://www.hrc.org/familynet/chapter.asp?chapter$eq75>, accessed 9 January 2003.

Hunter, Nan D. 1997 [1991]. "Sexual Dissent and the Family: The Sharon Kowalski Case." In *Reconstructing Gender: A Multicultural Anthology,* edited by Estelle Disch, 295–99. Mountain View, Calif.: Mayfield Publishing Company.

Huxley, Aldous. 1998 [1932]. *Brave New World.* New York: HarperPerennial.

International Federation of Fertility Societies. 1995. "International Consensus on Assisted Procreation." IFFS, Montpellier, France.

Inter-University Consortium for Political and Social Research (ICPSR): Social Science Data and Resources for Researchers. "National Survey of Family Growth (NSFG)

Series." <http://www.icpsr.umich.edu:8080/ICPSR-SERIES/00048.xml>, accessed 28 December 2002.

International Gay and Lesbian Human Rights Commission. 2003. "When Having Sex is a Crime: Criminalization and Decriminalization of Homosexual Acts (2003)." http://www.iglhrc.org/site/iglhrc/content.php?type=1&id=77#AZCountry, accessed 19 October, 2003.

————. 1998. "Registered Partnership, Domestic Partnership, and Marriage: A Worldwide Summary Compiled by the IGLHRC in November, 1998." <http://www .iglhrc.org/news/factsheets/marriage_981103.html>, accessed 28 June 2002.

Irigaray, Luce. 1985a. Speculum of the Other Woman. Ithaca, N.Y.: Cornell University Press.

————. 1985b. This Sex Which Is Not One. Ithaca, N.Y.: Cornell University Press.

Irvine, Janice M. 1990. Disorders of Desire: Sex and Gender in Modern American Sexology. Philadelphia: Temple University Press.

Jack, Rand, and Dana Crowley Jack. 1989. Moral Vision and Professional Decisions: The Changing Values of Women and Men Lawyers. Cambridge [England] and New York: Cambridge University Press.

Jacob, M.C., S.C. Klock, and D. Maier. 1999. "Lesbian Couples as Therapeutic Donor Insemination Recipients: Do They Differ from Other Patients?" Journal of Psychosomatic Obstetrics and Gynecology 20: 203–15.

Joffe, Carol. 1986. The Regulation of Sexuality: Experiences of Family Planning Workers. Philadelphia: Temple University Press.

Johnson, Suzanne M., and Elizabeth O'Connor. 2002. The Gay Baby Boom: The Psychology of Gay Parenthood. New York and London: New York University Press.

Jones, Jacqueline. 1985. Labor of Love, Labor of Sorrow: Black Women, Work, and the Family from Slavery to the Present. New York: Basic Books.

Kahn, Susan Martha. 2000. Reproducing Jews: A Cultural Account of Assisted Reproduction in Israel. Durham and London: Duke University Press.

Kalser, Denise S. 1987 1988. "Artificial Insemination: Donor Rights in Situations Involving Unmarried Recipients." Journal of Family Law 26: 793–811.

Kallen, Evelyn. 1996. "Gay and Lesbian Rights Issues: A Comparative Analysis of Sydney, Australia and Toronto, Canada." Human Rights Quarterly 18: 206–23.

Kaplan, E. Ann, and Susan Squier, eds. 1999. Playing Dolly: Technocultural Formations, Fantasies, and Fictions of Assisted Reproduction. New Brunswick, N.J.: Rutgers University Press.

Katz, Jonathan. 1995. The Invention of Heterosexuality. New York: Dutton.

Kendall, Kate, and Robert Haaland. 1996. Lesbians Choosing Motherhood: Legal Implications of Alternative Insemination and Reproductive Technologies. San Francisco: National Center for Lesbian Rights.

Kimbrell, Andrew. 1993. The Human Body Shop: The Engineering and Marketing of Life. San Francisco: Harper.

Klein, Renate Duelli. 1994. "Doing It Ourselves: Self-Insemination." In Test-Tube

Women: What Future for Motherhood? Edited by Rita Arditti, Renate Duelli Klein, and Shelley Minden, 382–390. London: Pandora Press.

Klock, S.C., M.C. Jacob, and D. Maier. 1996. "A Comparison of Single and Married Recipients of Donor Insemination." *Journal of Human Reproduction* 11: 2554–57.

Koehler, Kristin E. 1996. "Artificial Insemination: In the Child's Best Interest?" *Albany Law Journal of Science & Technology* 5: 321–23.

Koontz, Stephanie. 1997. *The Way We Really Are: Coming to Terms with America's Changing Families.* New York: Basic Books.

Kovacs, G.T., C.E. Clayton, and P. McGowan. 1983. "The Attitudes of Semen Donors." *Clinical Reproduction and Fertility* 2: 73–75.

Kramerae, Cheris, and Dale Spender, eds. 2000. *Routledge International Encyclopedia of Women: Global Women's Issues and Knowledge.* New York and London: Routledge.

Kritchevsky, Barbara, 1981. "The Unmarried Woman's Right to Artificial Insemination: A Call for an Expanded Definition of Family." *Harvard Women's Law Journal* 4, no. 1: 19.

Lacan, Jacques. 1977 [1953]. "The Significance of the Phallus." In *Ecrits: A Selection.* Translated by Alan Sheridan, 281–91. New York: W.W. Norton.

Lacey, Linda J. 1996. "Book Review: As American as Parenthood and Apple Pie: Neutered Mothers, Breadwinning Fathers, and Welfare Rhetoric." *Cornell Law Review* 82: 79–108.

Ladd-Taylor, Molly, and Lauri Umansky, eds. 1998. *"Bad" Mothers: The Politics of Blame in Twentieth-Century America.* New York: New York University Press.

Lash, Scott. 1990. *Sociology of Postmodernism.* London and New York: Routledge.

Lasker, Judith N. 1998. "The Users of Donor Insemination." In *Donor Insemination: International Social Science Perspectives,* edited by Ken Daniels and Erica Haimes, 7–32. Cambridge: University of Cambridge Press.

Latour, Bruno. 1993. *We Have Never Been Modern.* Translated by Catherine Porter. Cambridge: Harvard University Press.

Leiblum, S.R., M.G. Palmer, and I.P. Spector. 1995. "Non-Traditional Mothers: Single Heterosexual/Lesbian Women and Lesbian Couples Electing Motherhood via Donor Insemination." *Journal of Psychosomatic Obstetrics and Gynecology* 16: 11–20.

Lesbian Mom's Organization Webpage. 1995. "Laws Relating to AI/Adoption." http://www.lesbian.org/moms/law.htm. Accessed June 15, 1998.

Lévi-Strauss, Claude. 1967 [1958]. *Structural Anthropology.* New York: Doubleday Anchor. Translated by Claire Jacobson and Brooke Grundfest-Schoepf.

Lewin, Ellen. 1993. *Lesbian Mothers: Accounts of Gender in American Culture.* Ithaca, N.Y.: Cornell University Press.

———. 1994. "Negotiating Lesbian Motherhood: The Dialectic of Resistance and Accommodation." In *Mothering: Ideology, Experience, and Agency,* edited by E. Nakano Glenn, G. Chang, and L.R. Forcey, 333–53. New York: Routledge.

Lockman, Lawrence. 1999. "Psychologist Peter Rees Hates 'Homophobia,' But Can He Tell Us What It Is?" In *As Maine Goes,* 24 March.

<http://www.asmainegoes.com/Columnists/Lockman/lockman14.htm>, accessed 18 July 2002.

Lorde, Audre. 1984. *Sister Outsider: Essays and Speeches.* Trumansburg, N.Y.: Crossing Press.

Lui, S.C., S.M. Weaver, J. Robinson, M. Debono, M. Nieland, S.R. Killick, and D.M. Hay. 1995. "A Survey of Semen Donor Attitudes." *Human Reproduction* 10: 234–38.

Lynch, Margaret A., and Richard S. Ferri. 1997. "Health Needs of Lesbian Women and Gay Men: Providing Quality Care." *Clinician Reviews* 7, no. 1: 85–118.

Macaulay, L., J. Kitzinger, G. Green, and D. Wight. 1995. "Unconventional Conceptions and HIV." *AIDS Care* 3, no. 7: 261–76.

MacCannell, Juliet Flower. 1991. *The Regime of the Brother: After the Patriarchy.* New York and London: Routledge.

Macdonald, Cameron L. 1992. "Nuclear Family Fissions: Reproductive Technologies, Parental Rights, and Judicial Decision Making." Unpublished Paper. Author's personal collection.

MacKinnon, Catherine. 1991 [1983]. "Feminism, Marxism, Method, and the State." In *Feminist Legal Theory: Readings in Law and Gender,* edited by K.T. Bartlett, and Rosanne Kennedy, 181–200. Boulder, San Francisco, and Oxford: Westview Press.

———. 1996. "Law's Stories as Reality and Politics." In *Law's Stories: Narrative and Rhetoric in the Law,* edited by P. Brooks and Paul Gewirtz, 232–37. New Haven and London: Yale University Press.

Mamo, Laura. 2002. *Sexuality, Reproduction, and Biomedical Negotiations: An Analysis of Achieving Pregnancy in the Absence of Heterosexuality.* Doctoral dissertation, University of California, San Francisco.

Mankiller, Wilma, Gwendolyn Mink, Marysa Navarro, Barbara Smith, and Gloria Steinem, eds. 1998. *The Reader's Companion to U.S. Women's History.* Boston and New York: Houghton Mifflin Company.

Mann, Paul. 1995. "Stupid Undergrounds." *Postmodern Culture* 5.

Markowitz, Deborah L., "The Vermont Guide to Civil Unions." State of Vermont, Office of the Secretary of the state. <http://www.sec.state.vt.us/otherprg/civilunions/civilunions.html>, accessed 24 June 2002.

Marquis, Julie. 2000. "Court Limits Anonymity of Sperm Donors." *Los Angeles Times,* 20 May 2000. <http://www.latimes.com/news/state/20000520/t000047636.html>, accessed 30 May 2000.

Martin, April. 1993. *The Lesbian and Gay Parenting Handbook: Creating and Raising Our Families.* New York: HarperPerennial.

Martin, Emily. 1999. "The Woman in the Flexible Body." In *Revisioning Women, Health and Healing: Feminist, Cultural, and Technoscience Perspectives,* edited by Adele E. Clarke and Virginia L. Olesen, 97–115. New York: Routledge.

Massey, Alexander. 1999. "Methodological Triangulation, Or How to Get Lost without Being Found Out." In *Explorations in Methodology, Studies in Educational Ethnography,* vol. 2, edited by A. Massey and G. Walford, 183–97. Stamford, Conn.: JAI Press.

Masters, William, and Virginia Johnson. 1966. *Human Sexual Response.* New York: Bantam Books.

Mattes, Jane. 1994. *Single Mothers by Choice: A Guidebook for Single Women Who Are Considering or Have Chosen Motherhood.* New York: Times Books/Random House.

Mauss, Marcel. 1967 [1925]. *The Gift: Forms and Functions of Exchange in Archaic Societies.* Translated by Ian Cunnison. New York: W.W. Norton.

McCarrick, Pat Milmoe. 1996. "Feminist Perspectives on Bioethics." *Kennedy Institute of Ethics Journal* 6: 85–103.

McKinlay, John B., and J. Arches. 1985. "Towards the Proletarianization of Physicians." *The International Journal of Health Services* 15, no. 2: 161–95.

McKinlay, John B., and John D. Stoeckle. 2001 [1988]. "Corporatization and the Social Transformation of Doctoring." In *The Sociology of Health and Illness: Critical Perspectives,* sixth edition, edited by Peter Conrad, 175–86. New York: Worth Publishers.

Millbank, Jenni. 1996. "An Implied ??MS 366 Pronyx?? to Prevent: Lesbian Families, Litigation and W v G (1996) 20 Fam LR 49." *Australian Journal of Family Law* 10: 112.

Miller, Alice M., AnnJanette Rosga, and Meg Satterthwaite. 1999. "Health, Human Rights, and Lesbian Existence." In *Health and Human Rights: A Reader,* edited by Jonathan M. Mann, Sofia Gruskin, Michael A. Grodin, and George J. Annas, 265–80. New York and London: Routledge.

Miller, Naomi. 1992. *Single Parents by Choice: A Growing Trend in Family Life.* New York and London: Insight Books/Plenum Press.

Minow, Martha. 1991. "Redefining Families: Who's In and Who's Out?" *University of Colorado Law Review* 62: 269–85.

———. 1993. *Family Matters: Readings on Family Life and the Law.* New York: The New Press.

Minter, Shannon. 1996. "United States." In *Unspoken Rules: Sexual Orientation and Women's Human Rights,* edited by R. Rosenbloom, and the International Commission for Gay and Lesbian Human Rights, 209–21. London and New York: Cassell.

Mohler, Marie, and Lacy Frazer. 2002. *A Donor Insemination Guide: Written by and for Lesbian Women.* Binghamton, N.Y.: Alice Street Editions.

Moraga, Cherríe. 1997. *Waiting in The Wings: Portrait of a Queer Motherhood.* Ithaca, N.Y.: Firebrand Books.

Morgan, Kathryn Pauly. 1996. "The Moral Politics of Sex Education." In *The Gender Question in Education: Theory, Pedagogy, and Politics,* by Ann Diller, Barbara Houston, Kathryn Pauly Morgan, and Maryann Ayim, with a forward by Jane Roland Martin, 170–78. Boulder and Oxford: Westview Press.

Mossman, Mary Jane. 1991. "Feminism and Legal Method: The Difference it Makes." In *At the Boundaries of the Law: Feminism and Legal Theory,* edited by Martha Albertson Fineman and Nancy Sweet Thomadsen, 283–300. New York and London: Routledge.

Murphy, Julien S. 2001. "Should Lesbians Count as Infertile Couples? Anti-Lesbian Discrimination in Assisted Reproduction." In *Queer Families, Queer Politics: Challeng-*

ing Culture and the State, edited by Mary Bernstein and Renate Reimann, 182–200. New York: Columbia University Press.

Nachtigall, R.D. 1993. "Secrecy: An Unresolved Issue in the Practice of Donor Insemination." *American Journal of Obstetrics and Gynecology* 168: 1846–49.

———. 1994. "Donor Insemination and Human Immunodeficiency Virus: A Risk/ Benefit Analysis." *American Journal of Obstetrics and Gynecology* 170, no. 6: 1692–96.

National Center for Lesbian Rights. 1991–1992. "Our Day In Court—Against Each Other: Intra-community Disputes Threaten All of Our Rights." *NCLR Newsletter* (Winter).

———. 1996. *State by State Guide to Child Custody.* San Francisco: National Center for Lesbian Rights.

———. 2001. "Second Parent Adoption, An Information Sheet." San Francisco: NCLR. Updated 16 July 2001.

———. 2003a. "Partnership Protection Documents." <http://www.nclrights.org/ publications/ppd.htm>, accessed 9 January 2003.

———. 2003b. "Second Parent Adoptions: A Snapshot of Current Law." <http://www .nclrights.org/publications/2ndparentadoptions.htm>, accessed November 11, 2003.

National Gay and Lesbian Task Force. "Specific Anti-Same-Sex Marriage Laws in the U.S.—June 2001." <http://www.ngltf.org/downloads/marriagemap0601.pdf>, accessed 28 June 2002.

———. "Adoption/Foster Care Laws in the U.S.—April 2002. <http://www.ngltf.org/ downloads/adoptionmap0402.pdf>, accessed 28 June 2002.

Nestle, Joan. 1987. *A Restricted Country.* Ithaca, N.Y.; Firebrand.

Nietzsche, Friedrich Wilhelm, Walter Arnold Kaufmann, and R.J. Hollingdale. 1968. *The Will to Power.* Translated by Der Wille zur Macht. New York: Vintage Books.

Noble, Elizabeth. 1987. *Having Your Baby by Donor Insemination: A Complete Resource Guide.* Boston: Houghton Mifflin Company.

Nordenberg, Tamar. 1997. "Science and ART." *FDA Consumer* (January/February).

Norsigian, Judy. 1976. "Proceedings for the 1975 Conference on Women and Health," 4–7 April 1975, Boston.

Nsiah-Jefferson, Laurie. 1994. "Reproductive Genetic Services for Low-Income Women and Women of Color: Access and Sociocultural Issues." In *Women and Prenatal Testing: Facing the Challenges of Genetic Technology,* edited by Karen H. Rothenberg and Elizabeth J. Thomson, 234–59. Columbus: Ohio State University Press.

O'Brien, Mary. 1981. *The Politics of Reproduction.* London: Routledge & Kegan Paul Ltd.

O'Hanlan, Kate. 1995. "Lesbian Health and Homophobia: Perspectives for the Treating Obstetrician/Gynecologist." *Current Problems in Obstetrics, Gynecology, and Fertility* 4: 97–133.

Okun, Barbara F., Jane Fried, and Marcia L. Okun. 1999. *Understanding Diversity: A Learning-as-Practice Primer.* Pacific Grove, Calif.: Brooks-Cole Publishing.

O'Neill, John. 1985. *Five Bodies: The Human Shape of Modern Society.* Ithaca and London: Cornell University Press.

Overall, Christine. 1987. *Ethics and Human Reproduction: A Feminist Analysis.* Boston: Allen and Unwin.

Pacific Reproductive Services (PRS). 1997. "Information Package." San Francisco: PRS.

———. 2002a. "Becoming a Sperm Donor," <http://www.hellobaby.com/bedonor.html>, accessed 21 June 2002.

———. 2002b. "April 2002 Donor Catalogue." <http://www.hellobaby.com/profiles.html>, accessed 7 August 2002.

Pateman, Carole. 1988. *The Sexual Contract.* London: Polity Press.

Patterson, Charlotte J. 1992. "Children of Lesbian and Gay Parents." *Child Development* 63: 1025–42.

———. 1995. "Families of the Lesbian Baby Boom: Parents' Division of Labor and Children's Adjustment. *Developmental Psychology* 31, no. 1: 115–23.

Paul, Diane B. 1995. *Controlling Human Heredity: 1865 to the Present.* Atlantic Highlands, N.J.: Humanities Press International.

Pepper, Rachel. 1999. *The Ultimate Guide to Pregnancy for Lesbians: Tips and Techniques from Conception through Birth: How to Stay Sane and Care for Yourself.* San Francisco: Cleis Press.

Perkoff, Gerald T. 1985. "Artificial Insemination in a Lesbian: A Case Analysis." *Annals of Internal Medicine* 145: 527.

Perspective Queer Parents (PQP). 1997. <http://www.geocities.com/WestHollywood/3373/>, accessed 28 August 1997.

———. 2002. "Perspective Queer Parents Ads." <http://www.queerparents.org/ads.html>, accessed 21 June 2002.

Petchesky, Rosalind Pollack. 1987. "Foetal Images: The Power of Visual Culture in the Politics of Abortion." In *Reproductive Technologies: Gender, Motherhood, and Medicine: Feminist Perspectives,* edited by Michelle Stanworth, 57–80. Minneapolis: University of Minnesota Press.

Pfeffer, Naomi. 1987. "Artificial Insemination, In-vitro Fertilization and the Stigma of Infertility." In *Reproductive Technologies: Gender, Motherhood and Medicine, Feminist Perspectives,* edited by Michelle Stanworth, 81–97. Minneapolis: University of Minnesota Press.

Pfeufer Kahn, Robbie. 1995. *Bearing Meaning: The Language of Birth.* Urbana: University of Illinois Press.

Pfohl, Stephen J. 1992. *Death at the Parasite Cafe: Social Science (Fictions) and the Postmodern.* Houndmills, Basingstoke, Hampshire: Macmillan.

Pies, Cheri. 1985. *Considering Parenthood: A Workbook for Lesbians.* San Francisco: Spinsters/Aunt Lute.

Pies, Cheri, and Francine Hornstein 1988. "Baby M & The Gay Family." *Out/Look:* 79–85.

Polikoff, Nancy D. 1987. "Lesbians Choosing Children: The Personal Is Political, Revisited." In *Politics of the Heart: A Lesbian Parenting Anthology,* edited by Sandra Pollack and Jeanne Vaughn, 51–53. Ithaca, N.Y.: Firebrand Books.

———. 1990. "This Child Does Have Two Mothers: Redefining Parenthood to Meet

the Needs of Children in Lesbian–Mother and Other Nontraditional Families."
Georgetown Law Journal 78: 459–575.

———. 1996. "The Deliberate Construction of Families without Fathers: Is it an Option for Lesbian and Heterosexual Mothers?" *Santa Clara Law Review* 36: 375–94.

Pollack, Sandra, and Jeanne Vaughn, eds. 1987. *Politics of the Heart: A Lesbian Parenting Anthology.* Ithaca, N.Y.: Firebrand Books.

Pollitt, Katha. 1996. "Don't Say I Didn't Warn You." In *Same-Sex Marriage: Pro and Con: A Reader,* edited by Andrew Sullivan, 196–99. New York: Vintage Books/Random House.

Pollock, Anne. 1998. "The Queers at the Center of High-Tech Reproduction: A Lesbian Body Sells Her Eggs." *critical in Queeries* 2, no. 1: 59–68.

———. In press. "Complicating Power in High-Tech Reproduction: Narratives of Anonymous Paid Egg Donors." *Journal of the Medical Humanities.*

Post, Dianne. 1997. "Why Marriage Should Be Abolished." *Women's Rights Law Reporter* 18: 283–312.

Poster, Mark. 1990. *The Mode of Information: Poststructuralism and Social Context.* Chicago: University of Chicago Press.

Prager, Susan Westerberg. 1982. "Shifting Perspectives on Marital Property Law." In *Rethinking the Family: Some Feminist Questions,* edited by B Thorne with M. Yalom, 111–30. New York and London: Longman.

Quebec, Canada. 2002. National Assembly, Second Session, Thirty-Sixth Legislature. *An Act instituting civil unions and establishing new rules of filiation,* no. 84, c. 6.

"Queers Read This," published anonymously by queers. First distributed at the New York City gay pride march, 1990. Author's collection.

Radicalesbians. 1973 [1970]. "The Woman Identified Woman." In *Radical Feminism,* edited by Anne Koedt, Ellen Levine, and Anita Rapone, 240–45. New York: Quadrangle.

Radin, Margaret Jane. 1996 *Contested Commodities.* Cambridge and London: Harvard University Press.

Rafkin, Louise. 1990. *Different Mothers: Sons and Daughters of Lesbians Talk about their Lives.* Pittsburgh and San Francisco: Cleis Press.

Rainbow Flag Health Services. 2002. "A Known Donor Sperm Bank." <http://www.gayspermbank.com>, accessed 21 June 2002.

Rapp, Rayna. 1982. "Family and Class in Contemporary America: Notes Toward an Understanding of Ideology." In *Rethinking the Family: Some Feminist Questions,* edited by B. Thorne with M. Yalom, 168–87. New York: Longman.

Rapping, Elayne. 1990. "The Future of Motherhood: Some Unfashionably Visionary Thoughts." In *Women, Class, and the Feminist Imagination,* edited by K. V. Hansen, and I.J. Philipson, 537–48. Philadelphia: Temple University Press.

Raymond, Janice G. 1993. *Women as Wombs: Reproductive Technologies and the Battle Over Women's Freedom.* San Francisco: HarperSanFrancisco.

Reinfeld, Moshe. 2000. "High Court: Child May Have Two Mothers." Ha'aretz News,

Internet edition. 30 May, 2000. http://www.nclrights.org/releases/haaretz.htm, accessed 19 October 2003.

Reproductive Technologies, Inc. 1997. "1997 TSBC Fee Schedule." Berkeley: The Sperm Bank of California.

Resolve. 2003. "Resolve: The National Infertility Association." <http://www.resolve.org>, accessed 18 July 2003.

Rich, Adrienne Cecile. 1976. *Of Woman Born: Motherhood as Experience and Institution*. New York: W.W. Norton and Company.

———. 1979 [1977]. "Husband-Right and Father-Right." In *On Lies, Secrets, and Silence: Selected Prose 1966–1978*. New York and London: W.W. Norton and Company.

———. 1979. *On Lies, Secrets, and Silence*. New York: W.W. Norton and Company.

———. 1981. *Compulsory Heterosexuality and Lesbian Existence*. London: Onlywomen Press.

———. 1986 [1980]. "Compulsory Heterosexuality and Lesbian Existence." In *Blood, Bread, and Poetry: Selected Prose 1979–1985*, 23–75. New York and London: W.W. Norton and Company.

Roberts, Dorothy E. 1997. "The Value of Black Mothers' Work." In *Critical Race Feminism: A Reader*, edited by A.K. Wing, 315–16. New York and London: New York University Press.

Robertson, John A. 1994. *Children of Choice: Freedom and the New Reproductive Technologies*. Princeton: Princeton University Press.

Robson, Ruthann. 1992. *Lesbian (Out)Law*. Ithaca, N.Y.: Firebrand Books.

———. 1995. "The Legal Domestication of Lesbian Existence." In *Mothers in Law: Feminist Theory and the Legal Regulation of Motherhood, Gender and Culture*, edited by M.A. Fineman and I. Karpin, 103–17. New York: Columbia University Press.

———. 1998. *Sappho Goes to Law School*. New York: Columbia University Press.

Rosenbloom, Rachel, ed. 1996. *Unspoken Rules: Sexual Orientation and Women's Human Rights*. London and New York: Cassell.

Ross, Thomas. 1996. *Just Stories: How the Law Embodies Racism and Bias*. Boston: Beacon Press.

Rothman, Barbara Katz. 1989. *Recreating Motherhood: Ideology and Technology in a Patriarchal Society*. New York and London: W.W. Norton and Company.

———. 1992. "The Frightening Future of Baby-Making: The New Reproductive Technologies May Turn Out To Be the Breast Implants of Tomorrow." *Glamour*, June 1992, 211–53.

Rothschild, Cynthia, edited and with contributions by Scott Long. 2000. *Written Out: How Sexuality Is Used to Attack Women's Organizing*. A report of the International Gay and Lesbian Human Rights Commission and the Center for Women's Global Leadership. San Francisco, California: IGLHRC.

Rotkin, Karen F. 1976. "The Phallacy of Our Sexual Norm." In *Beyond Sex-Role Stereotypes: Readings Toward a Psychology of Androgyny*, 154–62. Boston: Little, Brown, and Company. First published in *RT: A Journal of Radical Therapy* (formerly *Rough Times, Radical Therapist* 3, no. 1 (September 1972).

Rowland, Robyn. 1983. "Attitudes and Opinions of Donors on an Artificial Insemination by Donor (AID) Programme." *Clinical Reproduction and Fertility* 2: 249–59.

———. 1985. "The Social and Psychological Consequences of Secrecy in Artificial Insemination by Donor (AID) Programmes." *Social Science Medicine* 21: 391–96.

Rubin, Gayle. 1990 [1976]. "The Traffic in Women: Notes on the 'Political Economy' of Sex." In *Women, Class, and the Feminist Imagination: A Socialist-Feminist Reader,* edited by K.V. Hansen, and I.J. Philipson, 74–113. Philadelphia: Temple University Press.

Santa Cruz Women's Health Collective. 1979. *Lesbian Health Matters!* East Palo Alto, Calif.: Up Press.

Sauer, M.V., M.J. Gorrill, K.B. Zeffer, and M. Bustillo. 1989. "Attitudinal Survey of Sperm Donors to an Artificial Insemination Clinic." *Journal of Reproductive Medicine* 34: 362–64.

Saxton, Marsha, and Florence Howe, eds. 1987. *With Wings: An Anthology of Literature by and about Women with Disabilities.* New York: Feminist Press at the City University of New York.

Scandinavian Cryobank. 2003. "Full Catalogue." <http://www.scandinaviancryobank.com/donors.asp?sort=1&order=asc&subject=donors>, accessed 16 June 2003.

Schmidt, Matthew, and Lisa Jean Moore. 1998. "Constructing a 'Good Catch,' Picking a Winner: The Development of Technosemen and the Deconstruction of the Monolithic Male." In *Cyborg Babies: From Techno-Sex to Techno Tots,* edited by Robbie Davis-Floyd and Joseph Dumit, 21–39. New York and London: Routledge.

Schneider, Karen S. 1998. "Foster Mom." *People,* 23 March 1998, 122–28.

Shulman, Sarah. 2000. "Kate Kendall Wants Lesbians to Keep Their Promises." In *Home Fronts: Controversies in Nontraditional Parenting,* edited by Jess Wells, 69–86. Los Angeles: Alyson Publications.

Schultz, Marjorie Maguire. 1990. "Reproductive Technology and Intent-Based Parenthood: An Opportunity for Gender Neutrality." *Wisconsin Law Review* [vol]: 297.

Sedgwick, Eve Kosofsky. 1990. *Epistemology of the Closet.* Berkeley. University of California Press.

———. 1993. "How to Bring Your Kids Up Gay." In *Fear of a Queer Planet: Queer Politics and Social Theory,* edited by Michael Warner, 69–81. Minneapolis and London: University of Minnesota Press.

Seidman, Steven. 1997. *Difference Troubles: Queering Social Theory and Sexual Politics.* Cambridge: Cambridge University Press.

Shapiro, E. Donald, and Lisa Schultz. 1985–1986. "Single Sex Families: The Impact of Birth Innovation upon Traditional Notions." *Journal of Family Law* 24: 271–81.

Sherman, Suzanne, ed. 1992. *Lesbian and Gay Marriage: Private Commitments, Public Ceremonies.* Philadelphia: Temple University Press.

Silliman, Yael, and Anannaya Bhattacharjee, eds. 2002. *Policing the National Body: Race, Gender, and Criminalization.* A Project of the Committee on Women, Population, and the Environment. Cambridge, Mass.: South End Press.

Slaughter, M.M. 1995. "Fantasies: Single Mothers and Welfare Reform" (Review of *The Neutered Mother, the Sexual Family, and Other Twentieth Century Tragedies*). *Columbia Law Review* 95: 2156–92.

Solinger, Rickie. 1998. "Poisonous Choice." In *"Bad" Mothers: The Politics of Blame in Twentieth-Century America,* edited by Molly Ladd-Taylor and Lauri Umansky, 318–402. New York: New York University Press.

Sperm Bank Directory.Com. 2002. <www.spermbankdirectory.com>, accessed 31 August 2002.

Sperm Bank of California, The 2003. "Sperm Donor Catalogue." <http://www. thespermbankofca.org/catalog/indexc.htm>, accessed 4 November 2003.

Stacey, Judith. 1996. *In the Name of the Family: Rethinking Family Values in the Postmodern Age.* Boston: Beacon Press.

Stacey, Judith, and Timothy J. Biblarz. 2001. "(How) Does the Sexual Orientation of Parents Matter?" *American Sociological Review* 66: 159–83.

Stacey, Judith, and Elizabeth Davenport. 2002. "Queer Families Quack Back." In *Handbook of Lesbian and Gay Studies,* edited by Diane Richardson, 355–74. Thousand Oaks, Calif.: Sage Publications.

Stack, Carol B. 1974. *All Our Kin: Strategies for Survival in a Black Community.* New York: BasicBooks.

Staff, Dispatch-Reuters. 1997. "Lesbian to Pay Child Support." <http://www.glaad. org/glaad/dispatch/0603/07.html>, accessed 26 June 1997.

Staff, Drug Benefit Trends. 1997. "Current Health Care Events: Newsbriefs Index." *Drug Benefit Trends* 9: 11–18.

Stanworth, Michelle. 1987. *Reproductive Technologies: Gender, Motherhood and Medicine.* Minneapolis: University of Minnesota Press.

———. 1990. "Birth Pangs: Conceptive Technologies and the Threat to Motherhood." In *Conflicts in Feminism,* edited by M. Hirsch, and E. Fox Keller, 288–304. New York and London: Routledge.

Stein, Arlene. 1997. *Sex and Sensibility: Stories of a Lesbian Generation.* Berkeley, Los Angeles, and London: University of California Press.

Stephenson, Patricia St. Clair, and Marsden G. Wagner. 1991. "Turkey-baster Babies: A View from Europe." *Milbank Quarterly* 69: 45–50.

Stern, Judy E., Catherine P. Cramer, Andrew Garrod, and Ronald M. Green. 2001. "Access to Services at Assisted Reproductive Technology Clinics: A Survey of Policies and Practices." *American Journal of Obstetrics and Gynecology,* 184, no. 4: 591–97.

Strathern, Marilyn. 1992. *Reproducing the Future: Anthropology, Kinship, and the New Reproductive Technologies.* New York: Routledge.

Strong, C., and J.S. Schinfeld. 1984. "The Single Woman and Artificial Insemination by Donor." *Journal of Reproductive Medicine* 29, no. 5: 293–99.

Stychin, Carl, and Didi Herman, eds. 1995. *Legal Inversions: Lesbians, Gay Men, and the Politics of Law.* Philadelphia: Temple University Press.

Sullivan, Andrew. 1997. *Same-Sex Marriage: Pro and Con: A Reader.* New York: Vintage Books/Random House.

Sullivan, Maureen. 1996. "Rozzie and Harriet? Gender and Family Patterns of Lesbian Coparents." *Gender and Society* 10, no. 6: 747–67.

Sullivan, Ronald. 1992. "Judge Allows for Adoption by Lesbian: Says Gay Relationship Can't Block Procedure," *New York Times* 31 January, 416.

Teish, Louisa. 1985. *Jambalaya: The Natural Woman's Book of Personal Charms and Practical Rituals.* San Francisco: Harper and Row.

Terry, Jennifer. 1995. "Anxious Slippages between 'Us' and 'Them': A Brief History of the Scientific Search for Homosexual Bodies." In *Deviant Bodies: Critical Perspectives on Difference in Science and Popular Culture, Race, Gender, and Science,* edited by J. Urla and J. Terry, 129–69. Bloomington and Indianapolis: Indiana University Press.

———. 1997. "The Seductive Power of Science in the Making of Deviant Subjectivity." In *Science and Homosexualities,* edited by Vernon Rosario, 271–95. New York and London: Routledge.

Terry, Jennifer, and Jacqueline Urla. 1995. "Deviant Bodies: Critical Perspectives on Difference in Science and Popular Culture." In *Race, gender, and science,* 416. Bloomington: Indiana University Press.

Testy, Kelley Y. 1995. "An Unlikely Resurrection." *Northwestern University Law Review* 90: 219–35.

Theweleit, Klaus. 1987 [1977]. *Male Fantasies,* Volume One: *Women, Floods, Bodies, History.* Translated by Stephen Conway in collaboration with Erica Carter and Chris Turner. Minneapolis: University of Minnesota.

———. 1989. *Male Fantasies,* Volume Two: *Male Bodies—Psychoanalyzing the White Terror.* Translated by Chris Turner in collaboration with Erica Carter. Minneapolis: University of Minnesota.

Thompson, Becky. 1994. *A Hunger So Wide and So Deep: American Women Speak Out on Eating Problems.* Minneapolis. University of Minnesota Press.

Thorne, Barrie. 1993. *Gender Play: Girls and Boys in School.* New Brunswick N.J.: Rutgers University Press.

Todd, Alexandra Dundas. 1989. *Intimate Adversaries: Cultural Conflict between Doctors and Women Patients.* Philadelphia: University of Pennsylvania Press.

Traiman, Leland. 1998. "A Known Donor Sperm Bank Serving the Gay and Lesbian Community of the San Francisco Bay Area." Rainbow Flag Health Services. <http://www.flash.net/~rainbowf>, accessed 21 August 1997.

Trinh, T. Minh-Ha. 1989. *Woman, Native, Other: Writing Postcoloniality and Feminism.* Bloomington: Indiana University Press.

TSBC. 1997. "Information Package." <http://www.thespermbankofca.org>. Berkeley: Reproductive Technologies, Inc.

———. 2002a. <http://www.thespermbankofca.org/services/indexs.htm>, accessed 21 June 2002.

———. 2002b. "Our Mission Statement," <http://www.thespermbankofca.org/aboutus/indexa.htm>, accessed 21 June 2002.

———. 2002c. "Sperm Donor Catalogue: April–June 2002," <http://www.thespermbankofca.org/catalog/indexc.htm>, accessed 21 June 2002.

———. 2002d. "Sperm Donor Catalogue: July–September 2002," <http://www.thespermbankofca.org/catalog/indexc.htm>, accessed 15 August 2002.

Tsing, Anna Lowenhaupt. 1990. "Monster Stories: Women Charged with Perinatal Endangerment." In *Uncertain Terms: Negotiating Gender in American Culture*, edited by Faye Ginsburg, and Anna Lowenhaupt Tsing, 282–99. Boston: Beacon Press.

U.S. Census Bureau. 1997. "Child Support—Award and Recipiency Status of Custodial Parent: 1997. *Statistical Abstract of the United States*, no. 547.

U.S. Congress, Office of Technology Assessment. 1988. *Artificial Insemination: Practice in the United States: Summary of a 1987 Survey—Background Paper*, OTA-13P-BA-48. Washington D.C.: U.S. Government Printing Office, August.

Vagelatos, John. 1995. "Heeding Cassandra: The Neutered Mother, the Sexual Family, and Other Twentieth Century Tragedies." *Columbia Journal of Women and Law* 5: 127–41.

Vanfraussen, K., I. Ponjaert-Kristoffersen, and A. Brewaeys. 2001. "An Attempt to Reconstruct Children's Donor Concept: A Comparison between Children's and Lesbian Parents' Attitudes Towards Donor Anonymity." *Human Reproduction* 16, no. 9: 2019–25.

Vizenor, Gerald. 1990. "Socioacupuncture: Mythic Reversals and the Striptease in Four Acts." In *Out There: Marginalization and Contemporary Culture*, edited by R. Ferguson, Martha Gever, Trinh T. Minh-ha, and Cornel West, 411–19. New York, Cambridge, and London: The New Museum of Contemporary Art and the MIT Press.

Wakeling, Louise, and Margaret Bradstock. 1995. *Beyond Blood: Writings on the Lesbian and Gay Family.* Sydney, Australia: BlackWattle Press.

Walters, Leroy. 1996. "Current and Future Issues in Assisted Reproduction." *Kennedy Institute of Ethics Journal* 6: 383–87.

Warner, Michael, ed. 1993. *Fear of a Queer Planet: Queer Politics and Social Theory.* Minneapolis and London: University of Minnesota Press.

Watney, Simon. 1990. "Missionary Positions: AIDS, 'Africa,' and Race." In *Out There: Marginalization and Contemporary Cultures*, edited by M.G. Russell Fergusen, Trinh T. Minh-ha, and Cornel West, 89–103. New York, Cambridge, and London: The New Museum of Contemporary Art and The MIT Press.

Wegar, Katarina. 1997. *Adoption, Identity, and Kinship.* New Haven and London: Yale University Press.

Wehr, Mark. 2002. "Contemporary Theory." <http://www.ssc.wisc.edu/~kwehr/248lect4.pdf>, accessed 29 December 2002.

Wells, Jess, ed. 1997. *Lesbians Raising Sons: An Anthology.* Boston: Alyson Publications.

Wendland, C.L., F. Burn, and C. Hill. 1996. "Donor Insemination: A Comparison of Lesbian Couples, Heterosexual Couples and Single Women." *Fertility and Sterility* 65: 764–70.

Wertz, Richard W., and Dorothy C. Watz. 1989. *Lying-In: A History of Childbirth in America.* New Haven and London: Yale University Press.

West, Robin. 1991 [1988]. "Jurisprudence and Gender." In *Feminist Legal Theory: Readings in Law and Gender,* edited by K. T. Bartlett, and R. Kennedy, 201–34. Boulder, San Francisco, and Oxford: Westview Press.

Weston, Kath. 1991. *Families We Choose: Lesbians, Gays, Kinship.* New York: Columbia University Press.

———. 1996. *Render Me, Gender Me: Lesbians Talk Sex, Class, Color, Nation, Studmuffins.* New York: Columbia University Press.

———. 1998 [1995]. "Theory, Theory, Who's Got the Theory? Or Why I'm Tired of That Tired Debate." In *Long Slow Burn: Sexuality and Social Science.* New York and London: Routledge.

White, Evelyn C. 1990. *The Black Women's Health Book: Speaking for Ourselves.* Seattle: The Seal Press.

Wikler, D. 1991. "Turkey-Baster Babies: The Demedicalization of Artificial Insemination." *Milbank Quarterly* 69: 5–40.

Williams, Patricia J. 1991. *The Alchemy of Race and Rights: Diary of a Law Professor.* Cambridge and London: Harvard University Press.

———. 1992. "A Rare Case Study of Muleheadedness and Men, or How to Try an Unruly Black Witch, with Excerpts from the Heretical Testimony of Four Women, Known to Be Hysterics, Speaking in Their Own Voices, as Translated for This Publication by Brothers Hatch, Simpson, DeConcini, and Specter." In *Race-ing Justice, En-gendering Power: Essays on Anita Hill, Clarence Thomas, and the Construction of Social Reality,* edited and with an introduction by Toni Morrison, 159–71.

———. 1995. *The Rooster's Egg: On the Persistence of prejudice.* Cambridge: Harvard University Press.

Wittig, Monique. 1990 [1980]. "The Straight Mind." In *Out There: Marginalization and Contemporary Cultures,* edited by R. Ferguson, Martha Gever, Trinh T. Minh-ha, and Cornel West, 51–58. New York, Cambridge and London: The New Museum of Contemporary Art and The MIT Press.

Woodhouse, Barbara Bennett. 1993. "Hatching the Egg: A Child-Centered Perspective on Parents' Rights." *Cordozo Law Review* 14: 1748–1806.

———. 2001. "Children's Rights." University of Pennsylvania Law School, Public Law Working Paper No. 06.

Woolf, Linda M. 2002. "Homohatred: Intersection of Sexism, Misogyny and Violence" <http://www.webster.edu/~woolflm/homohatred.html>, accessed 29 December 2002.

World Health Organization (WHO). 1993. "CID." Chapter V, code 302.

Wortley, Pascale M., Teresa A. Hammett, and Patricia L. Fleming. 1998. "Donor Insemination and Human Immunodeficiency Virus Transmission." *Obstetrics and Gynecology* 91, no. 4: 515–18.

Xytex. 2003. "Internet Donor Listing." <http://www.thespermbankofca.org/catalog/indexc.htm>, accessed 16 June 2003.

———. 2003a. "I.N.F.O./OPEN: Informative Narrated Fone Options (One-to-One)." <http://www.xytex.com/info.asp>, accessed 16 June 2003.

Zola, Irving K. 1990. "Medicine as an Institution of Social Control." In *The Sociology of Health and Illness: Critical Perspectives,* edited by P. Conrad, and Rochelle Kern, 398–408. New York: St. Martin's.

Zolbrod, Aline. 1988. "The Emotional Distress of the Artificial Insemination Patient." *Medical Psychotherapy* 1: 161–72.

ZyGen Laboratory. 1997. "Services and Fees Schedule." Van Nuys, Calif.: ZyGen Laboratory.

Index

Acupuncture, 173–74

Adoption: in Northern European law, 78, 79; psychosocial and identity issues of, 118, 208n.16; semen donation compared with relinquishing children for, 21. *See also* Second-parent adoption

AI. *See* Alternative insemination

AIDS: and frozen sperm, 196n.19; and gay men as sperm donors, 100, 115, 209n.25; and lesbian coalitions with gay men, 113–15; medical screening for, x, 188n.5; and regulation of AI, 73, 74, 202n.32; and self-insemination, 95–96, 195n.18

Alabama, 6–7

Alaska, 46

Alison D. v. Virginia M., 85

Alternative insemination (AI), 181; American Society of Reproductive Medicine guideline for, 55; assumptions about families challenged by, 1; and commodification of semen, 24, 26, 100–105; as conceptive technology, 183; consenting husband as legal father, 73, 82, 201n.29; continuum of regulation of, 11; costs of, 93–99; in disaggregation of motherhood and fatherhood, 8; doctors once having monopoly on, ix; enhancements to, 93, 94; eugenic implications of, 30, 31; the family and regulation of, 10–11; in "fertility medicine," 3; heterol-

ogous, 45; heterosexism of, 7; homologous, 45; husband's consent for, 69, 73, 82, 201n.29; and infertility, 43–46; insurance coverage for, 46–47; intracytoplasmic sperm injection reducing market for, xi; legal regulation of, 11, 58–59, 68–69, 73–74, 199n.8; medicalization of, x, 38, 53, 115; in National Survey of Family Growth, 52; nuclear family as basis of, 2, 3, 6, 7, 27; paternalist resistance to, 24–26; physicians' gatekeeper role in, ix, 5; as product of its historical and ideological context, 35; in Quebec civil union law, 78; restricting to physicians, 5, 37, 74, 191n.15, 195n.4, 202n.33; secrecy regarding, 5–7, 191n.21; sexuality separated from procreation in, 106; social stratification in, 91, 93; statistics on, 4, 190n.12. *See also* Lesbian alternative insemination

American Civil Liberties Union (ACLU), 84–85

American Society of Reproductive Medicine (ASRM), 30, 43, 48, 49, 55, 95, 100

Animal husbandry, 26, 193n.28

Anti-abortion movement, 192n.4

Anti-discrimination statutes, 141

Anzaldúa, Gloria, 35

Aptheker, Bettina, 184

Arkansas, 47, 70

ART. *See* Assisted reproductive technology

Artificial insemination: criticisms of term, 181.
  See also Alternative insemination
ASRM (American Society of Reproductive
  Medicine), 30, 43, 48, 49, 55, 95, 100
Assisted reproductive technology (ART):
  connotations of term, 182; social stratifica-
  tion in, 91–93. *See also* Contractual and
  technological procreation
Australia, 147

"Baby M." surrogacy case, 32–33
Bartlett, Katherine T., 81, 153–54
Belgium, 61, 119
Benson, Sandra, 62–63
Berner-Kadish, Ruthie and Nicole, 85–86
"Best interests of the child" standard, 127, 159,
  164
Biomedicine. *See* Medical profession
Birth certificates, 82, 85
Blank, Robert H., 11, 58–59
Blankenhorn, David, 25–26
Blood, 27–28; chosen kin versus blood ties,
  132–36. *See also* Kinship
Bonding, 84, 129, 169
Boston, x, 94
Boston Women's Health Collective, 39–40
Bottoms, Sharon, 77
Bowers v. Hardwick (1986), 8
Brave New World (Huxley), 182, 215n.13
Breadwinner, male, 208n.56
British Columbia, 62–63, 141

California, 47, 70–71, 73, 83, 86, 200n.17
California Cryobank, 126, 206n.12
Capitalist-patriarchy, 20–21
Carby, Hazel, 194n.54
Care: devaluation of, 90, 160; rights versus,
  150–53
Carrington, Christopher, 97, 98, 137, 138
Catholic Church, 27, 45–46, 193n.31, 207n.45
Centers for Disease Control and Prevention
  (CDCP), 5, 95
Chambers, David L., xiii, 13
Child custody: children's-rights approach and,
  165; lesbian co-mothers seeking, 146, 153;
  lesbian mothers challenged, 74–75, 77, 82,
  89, 125; maternal preference doctrine, 159;
  same-sex marriage and, 142; sperm donors
  seeking, 87
Children: "best interests of the child" standard,

127, 159, 164; children's-rights approach to
  the family, 163–66; of lesbian mothers, xiii,
  8; with multiple mothers, xvi; psychosocial
  importance of sperm donors, xi, 115–28;
  secondary dependency of, 157. *See also*
  Adoption; Child custody; Child support;
  Visitation
Children of Lesbians and Gays Everywhere
  (COLAGE), 124
Child support: AI codes cross-referenced to,
  73; fathers' abysmal record on, 163, 213n.56;
  by lesbian co-mothers, 74, 147; by sperm
  donors, 83
Citation, 177
Civil union, 69, 77–78, 141, 142
Cixous, Hélène, 206n.25
Class: in defining the family, 76; and "doing
  family," 93–99; in exploitation of women,
  102; stratification in infertility services, 91–
  92; stratification of sperm donors by, 100
Cloning, 24, 68, 183, 191n.23
Closet: lesbian mothers and the, 130–32, 167;
  power of the, 53
C. M. v. C. C. (1987), 68
Colen, Shellee, 205n.1
Colker, Ruth, 207n.32
Colorado, 200n.17
Coming out, lesbian mothers and, 130–32,
  167
Commodification, 23, 16, 21, 22–27, 100–105
"Commodities among Themselves" (Irigaray),
  106
Co-mothers. *See* Lesbian co-mothers
Conception Connection, 120, 121, 124
Conceptive technologies, 183–84. *See also*
  Alternative insemination
Conference on Women and Health (1975), 12
Connecticut, 47, 73, 200n.17
Conrad, Peter, 47
Contraceptive technologies, 183
Contracts, legally binding, 149–50, 152–53
Contractual and technological procreation,
  182–84; AI receiving little attention in
  debates on, 15; categories of, 183; centrality
  of lesbians to, 53, 56; commercialization of,
  100–101; debates over, 116; as dehumaniz-
  ing, 126; as stratified, 93. *See also* Alternative
  insemination
Convention on the Rights of the Child (1989),
  165–66

changes in, 78–79; in pre-modern family, 18; suppression of female identity in patriarchal, 45; transformation of, 8–9. *See also* Same-sex marriage

Maryland, 46

Massachusetts, 47, 147, 159, 200n.17

Masters, William, 212n.44

Matriarchal society, 194n.52

Mattes, Jane, 58

Medical profession: alternative, 187n.1; antihomophobic training for, 65; biomedical model, 37–38; changes in, ix–x, 5–7; commodification of health in, 47; on deviant women, 34–35; as discursive, xiv; elements of, 187n.1; the family and regulation of AI, 10–11; as instrument of social control, x, xiv, 5; lesbians' bad experiences with health care system, 99; as male-dominated, 37; medical anti-lesbianism, 57–61; physicians as gatekeepers in AI, ix, 5; physicians discriminating against single women, 141; physicians refusing to perform lesbian AI, ix, 54, 61, 62, 63, 83, 197n.53; restricting AI to physicians, 5, 37, 74, 191n.15, 195n.4, 202n.33; self-insemination contrasted with that by, 39–43. *See also* Infertility medicine

Medical screening, x, 12, 41, 93, 188n.5

Medicalization, x, xi, 38, 53, 115

Methodology of this study, 173–75

Military, lesbians and gay men in the, 142

Minnesota, 64

Minow, Martha, 82, 148, 156

Mintzer, Shannon, 77

Mississippi, 70

Mohler, Marie, 42

Montana, 47

Moore, Lisa Jean, 99–100

Moraga, Cherríe, 115

Morality laws, 72

Morgan, Kathryn Pauly, 202n.45

Motherhood: AI disaggregating fatherhood and, 8; in child custody cases, 159; in dependency-model of procreation, 169; "good" versus "bad" mothers, 33–35; lack of equivalence with fatherhood, 157–59; legal status of two mothers, 85–86; mother-child relationship for replacing marriage, 156–57; normative notions of family constraining, 77; patriarchy constraining, 171;

secondary dependency of mothers, 157, 160; surrogate motherhood, 1, 32–33, 43, 68, 84, 204n.74. *See also* Lesbian mothers; Single motherhood

Nachtigall, R. D., 95, 96

Names, 110

National Center for Lesbian Rights (NCLR), 67, 77, 96, 145

National Lesbian Family Study (NLFS), 118, 131, 132, 134

National Lesbian Rights Project, 64

National Survey of Family Growth (NSFG), 51–52, 91, 205n.4

Native Americans, 28

Nature: and blood, 27–28, 133; deviance as "unnatural," 88; lesbian appropriation of the "natural," 122; patriarchy "as natural," 16, 18, 170–71; in pre-modern conception of family, 16, 18, 87–88; same-sex eroticism "unnatural," 88–89, 128, 205n.87

NCLR (National Center for Lesbian Rights), 67, 77, 96, 145

Nebraska, 200n.17

Netherlands, the, 79, 203n.55

New Jersey, 47, 200n.17

New York State, 71, 85, 200n.17

NLFS (National Lesbian Family Study), 118, 131, 132, 134

Nobel Prize winners, 31

Nomos, 167–68, 169

Norway, 78

Nostalgia, 81, 128, 170–71, 204n.63

NSFG (National Survey of Family Growth), 51–52, 91, 205n.4

Nuclear family: AI as based on, 2, 3, 6, 7, 27, "breakdown" of, 128; demotion to one family form among many, 169; as "natural," 89. *See also* Male-dominated families

O'Brien, Mary, 18, 27

Office of Technology Assessment (OTA), 4, 5, 51–52, 192n.43, 197n.53

O'Hanlan, Kate, 13

Ohio, 200n.17

Oregon, 64

OTA (Office of Technology Assessment), 4, 5, 51–52, 192n.43, 197n.53

Outness, lesbian mothers and, 130–32, 167

Ova (egg) donation, 56–57, 157–58, 206n.30
Ovulation-prediction kits (OPK), x, 42, 94

Pacific Reproductive Services, 124, 206n.12
Pagan epistemologies, 175
Parents: de facto parents, 141, 142, 204nn. 72,
73; equitable parenthood, 154; in "functional" family, 84–85, 148–49, 154, 156;
gender-neutral parenting, 158; *in loco parentis,*
141; lesbian co-mothers' parental rights, 9,
67, 68, 69, 74, 83–86, 141, 142, 146–47; redefining parenthood, 153–55; sperm donors'
parental rights, 9, 21, 67, 68, 83, 87, 102,
141, 153. *See also* Fatherhood; Motherhood
Parthenogenesis, 171
Patriarchy: biological conception of fatherhood
in, 76; capitalist-patriarchy, 20–21; in legal
doctrine, xi, 82; lesbian AI as anti-patriarchal,
2, 105–10, 160–62, 168, 169; lesbian feminism resisting, 111, 112; in modern family,
18–19, 90, 193n.6; motherhood constrained
by, 171; names and, 110; as natural, 16, 18,
170–71; in pre-modern family, 16–18,
87–88, 89–90; semen valorized in, 23;
suppression of female identity in, 45; term
as used in this study, 188n.6. *See also*
Heteropatriarchy
Pennsylvania, 73, 200n.17
Pfeffer, Naomi, 24
Pfohl, Stephen, 189n.10
Phallus, the, 108–9
Physicians. *See* Medical profession
PIVMO, 76, 202n.45
Plato, 18, 27
Polikoff, Nancy, 154–55, 156, 166
"Political correctness," 113
Politics of the Heart: A Lesbian Parenting Anthology
(Pollack and Vaughn), 129–30
Pollock, Anne, 56–57, 206n.30
Postmodernity: lesbian AI as postmodern, 170;
postmodern family, 8–9, 17, 19–20, 135–36;
re-enchantment of lifeworld in, 23; shuffling
of signifiers in, 122; ultra-commodification
in, 103. *See also* Ultramodernity
Potter, Tracy, 62–63
Poverty, 43, 92, 213nn. 55, 56
Power-of-attorney agreements, 141
Precedent, legal, 81–82
Pregnancy: costs of achieving, 97; "flowerpot

model" of, 17–18, 27, 170, 192n.4; individ-
ualism contrasted with, 207n.38
Procreation. *See* Reproduction
Prospective Queer Parents (PQP), 119–21
Public accommodations laws, 141
Puerto Rico, 72, 73

Quebec, 77–78
Queer politics, 89, 113, 114
"Queers at the Center of High-Tech
Reproduction, The: A Lesbian Body Sells
Her Eggs" (Pollock), 56

Raboy, Barbara, 119
Race: blood as code word for, 28; in defining
the family, 76; interracial marriage, 211n.5;
and mother figure, 34, 194n.54; and queer
politics, 114; race-based labeling in sperm
banks, 31–32; as socio-political category, 32;
stratification in infertility services, 92–93;
stratification of sperm donors by, 100, 123
Radical strategies, 140
Rainbow Flag Health Services, 117, 122–23,
206n.12
Religion: Catholic Church, 27, 45–46,
193n.31, 207n.45; and gender equality, 108;
male supremacy justified by, 11; selecting
sperm donors by, 30; sin seen as unnatural,
88, 205n.86
Report of the National Survey of Family Growth,
51–52
Repository for Germinal Choice, 31
Reproduction (procreation): AI separating
sexuality from, 106; cloning, 24, 68, 183,
191n.23; dependency model of, 169–70;
parthenogenesis, 171; separation of social
from biological, 103–4; stratified, 91–93,
205n.1. *See also* Contractual and technological procreation; Pregnancy
Resemblance, 33, 194n.52
Rhode Island, 47
Rich, Adrienne, 11
Rights: care versus, 150–53; children's-rights
approach to the family, 163–66; human
rights, 52, 139, 142, 143, 164–66
Robson, Ruthann, xiv, 72–73, 98, 203n.45
Role models, 129
Roman Catholic Church, 27, 45–46, 193n.31,
207n.45

ABOUT THE AUTHOR

Amy Agigian is Associate Professor of Sociology at Suffolk University in Boston, where she is founder and director of the Center for Women's Health and Human Rights. She has been published in *Gender and Society, Disability Studies Quarterly,* and *Women's Studies International Forum.* She received her B.A. in Women's Studies and Comparative Religion from the University of California at Santa Cruz, and her M.A. and Ph.D. in Sociology from Brandeis University. She makes her home in Somerville, Massachusetts.